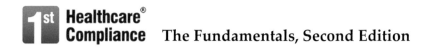

The Fundamentals, Second Edition

ISBN: 978-0-9991797-2-7

To order additional copies or to learn more about First Healthcare Compliance, call us at 888.54.FIRST (888.543.4778) or visit our website at www.1sthcc.com.

Table of Contents

Chapter 3

Chapter 4

Investigations and Remedial Measures

Discuss measures to mitigate ongoing harm: Physical security methods.

Physical security is essential for computer systems. The first step is to determine who should have access to different types of equipment and then to apply methods to limit access to those authorized through use of user names and passwords/tokens. Servers should be rack mounted and maintained in locked, climate-controlled rooms with regular surveillance.

Vulnerable devices should remain in the locked room. Data should be backed up routinely and stored/archived in a secure remote location. Workstations should be secure, including printers. Cable lock systems should be used to secure equipment, including laptops, to furniture. Operating systems should be locked when not in use and encryption software used to secure routers used for wireless transmission. Equipment should be in restricted areas. Remote access should be done with secure modems and encryption. Public access to the Internet should be on a different network from that used to transmit healthcare information.

Introduction

In 2012, nurse and attorney Julie Sheppard identified a widening gap between the expectations of government and the reality of healthcare compliance. Julie found that healthcare providers were becoming increasingly frustrated and intimidated by the increasing demands of complying with federal rules and regulations.

Julie's response was to launch First Healthcare Compliance to help physicians and other healthcare providers in private practice, hospital networks and health systems, healthcare billing companies and skilled nursing facilities comply with federal rules and regulations. After months of development, First Healthcare Compliance began offering its comprehensive healthcare compliance management solution in January 2013.

Since that time, First Healthcare Compliance has grown quickly to supply healthcare providers with a compliance management solution to help them avoid costly penalties, fines or more. Clients quickly discovered that the comprehensive program could help increase their staff communication, patient care and even improve the overall bottom line of their business.

In addition to its online component, First Healthcare Compliance offers valuable compliance resources, such as toll-free support, weekly blogs and newsletters, a webinar series, and most recently, an online fundamentals course for healthcare compliance. The online course covers the basics of HIPAA, OSHA, federal fraud and abuse laws and employment law.

Now in its second edition, this book serves as a companion guide to the online fundamentals course, although it can also be used as a stand-alone resource. The book is divided into four chapters, each addressing a critical healthcare compliance issue.

Chapter 1, Federal Healthcare Enforcement, provides a detailed discussion of fraud, waste and abuse practices as well as information about how to develop an effective compliance program to protect organizations from engaging in abusive practices and criminal activity.

Chapter 2, HIPAA, explores how the HIPAA Privacy, Security and Enforcement Rules impact healthcare providers, the key components of a HIPAA compliance plan, and the consequences of HIPAA noncompliance.

Chapter 3, OSHA, reviews the standards that healthcare employers must comply with, as well as the possible consequences of OSHA violations and a plan for compliance.

Chapter 4, Federal Employment Laws, considers the regulations that prohibit employee discrimination in recruiting, hiring, job evaluations, promotion policies, training, compensation and disciplinary action.

Each chapter includes a comprehensive list of online resources to provide readers with additional information.

This second edition provides updates to all four chapters, including a complete overhaul of the chapter on HIPAA.

We welcome your questions and the opportunity to assist you with additional resource materials and compliance services. Please don't hesitate to contact us with thoughts or questions.

The First Healthcare Compliance Team
888.54.FIRST
www.1sthcc.com

1st Healthcare® Compliance The Fundamentals, Second Edition *is designed to be an easy-to-understand, up-to-date reference to assist you with healthcare compliance concerns. However, this companion guide is not intended as legal advice, which will depend on facts, circumstances, and applicable law. The intricacies of this area of the law can result in serious penalties if a violation occurs. Readers should consider this book a starting point in this complex process and contact an attorney for legal advice, if needed.*

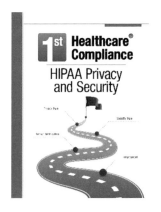

First Healthcare Compliance HIPAA Privacy and Security is a user-friendly resource designed to help healthcare, administrative, and compliance professionals, whether they serve as a covered entity or a business associate, better understand their compliance responsibilities under the Health Insurance Portability and Accountability Act. The book explains HIPAA privacy, security, enforcement and breach notification in plain language, and provides a comprehensive checklist that entities can use to get their compliance efforts off the ground.

About the Authors

Sheba Vine, JD, CIPP/US

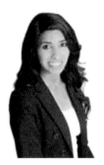

Sheba Vine is a lawyer and privacy professional that has written articles in the areas of privacy, human resource compliance, and healthcare laws. Sheba is certified by the International Association of Privacy Professionals (IAPP) as a Certified Information Privacy Professional (CIPP/US). Sheba worked in private practice, concentrating in litigation and employment laws. Prior to her legal career, Sheba held positions in the medical device industry with Hoffman La-Roche and Siemens. She received her Juris Doctorate from Widener University School of Law and her Bachelor of Science in Biomedical Engineering from Drexel University and is licensed to practice law in Delaware, New Jersey, Pennsylvania and before the U.S. Patent and Trademark Office.

Julie Sheppard BSN, JD, CHC
President and Founder, First Healthcare Compliance

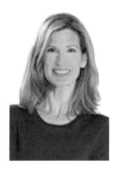

Julie Sheppard is a nurse, an attorney, and certified in Healthcare Compliance by the Compliance Certification Board. Married to a physician, her understanding of healthcare compliance issues grew from education, experience, and personal interest. With the increase in compliance challenges facing healthcare providers, Julie was inspired to create a practical, comprehensive healthcare compliance solution, and founded First Healthcare Compliance in 2012. Julie's professional memberships include the Pennsylvania Bar Association, the American Health Lawyers Association, and the Health Care Compliance Association.

About First Healthcare Compliance

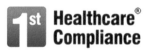

First Healthcare Compliance helps healthcare organizations of every size comply with an increasingly complex regulatory environment. Our software solution creates confidence among compliance professionals through education, resources, and support in the areas of HIPAA, OSHA, human resources compliance, and fraud waste and abuse laws. Serving clients across the United States, the company's evolving platform provides real-time insight for board reporting and across multiple locations. For more information please visit https://1sthcc.com/.

Chapter 1

Federal Healthcare Enforcement

Overview

In this chapter, you will learn how the federal government defines and enforces healthcare fraud and abuse practices. You will also learn how to develop a compliance program to protect your organization from engaging in abusive practices and criminal activity.

Chapter Outline

1.1   Understanding fraud, waste, and abuse
1.2   Federal fraud and abuse laws and enforcement agencies
1.3   The elements of an effective compliance program

Learning Objectives

After completing this chapter, you should be able to do the following:

✓   Describe and provide examples of the types of fraud, waste, and abuse that can occur in healthcare organizations.
✓   List the federal laws that address fraud, waste, and abuse.
✓   List the federal agencies responsible for enforcing healthcare fraud, waste, and abuse.
✓   Understand and explain the impact that fraud, waste and abuse can have on your organization.
✓   Describe the elements that an effective compliance program should have to help your organization avoid fraud, waste, and abuse.

1.1   Fraud, Waste, and Abuse

The abuse of federal healthcare programs like Medicare is a serious matter. Whether intentional or not, abusive practices like submitting excessive charges, billing for services not provided, or ordering unnecessary tests increases the financial strain on federal programs at a time when more and more of the population is served by them. They can also have serious consequences for providers found engaging in these activities.

 Fraudulent, wasteful and abusive practices create financial, regulatory and reputational risks for healthcare providers. Enforcement agencies may impose fines, exclusion from participation in federal programs or even criminal charges that can lead to imprisonment.

Federal laws define what constitutes fraud, waste, and abuse, as well as the penalties that a healthcare provider found guilty of these practices may face. Let's take a closer look at each topic.

1.1.1 Fraud

In the healthcare setting, fraud is defined as an intentional act of deception, misrepresentation, or concealment that is done in order to gain something of value. What does that mean?

Very simply, it means that a healthcare provider has knowingly made a false (fraudulent) claim to obtain a federal healthcare payment to which it is not entitled. Simpler still, it means the provider has lied about its services/activities in order to get money from the federal government.

What does healthcare fraud look like? Here are some examples:

- Billing for services not provided
- Billing for services at a higher rate than justified
- Soliciting, offering or receiving a kickback, bribe or rebate
- Violating the physician self-referral law

1.1.2 Waste

Waste is defined as "using or expending carelessly, extravagantly, or to no purpose." In the healthcare environment, waste is best understood as a form of mismanagement. A provider uses resources or spends money carelessly or fails to control costs, and then passes those excessive charges on to the federal government and to the taxpayers.

Unlike fraud, waste is not considered an intentional practice. The provider has not deliberately set out to deceive the federal government or misrepresent its activities. However, the outcome—overbilling the federal government—is the same, and it still carries consequences.

Here are some examples of waste:

- Providing services that are not medically necessary
- Performing tests or procedures that are not clinically indicated

1.1.3 Abuse

Abuse refers to intentional or unintentional practices that directly or indirectly result in unnecessary or increased costs to the Medicare program. It includes practices that are not "consistent with providing patients with services that are medically necessary, meet professionally recognized standards, and are priced fairly."

Examples of abuse in the healthcare setting include:

- Charging in excess for services or supplies

- Providing medically unnecessary services or providing services that do not meet professionally recognized standards

- Misusing codes on a claim, such as upcoding or unbundling codes

Fraud, waste, and abuse: What do they look like?

Fraud, waste, and abuse can occur anywhere in a healthcare provider's operations, including patient care, relationships with vendors and other service providers, and billing operations.

Here are a few scenarios that help illustrate fraud, waste, or abuse:

Prescription-related scenarios

Illegal remuneration schemes: A prescriber is offered, solicits, or receives money from a representative of a pharmaceutical or medical service or product provider in exchange for writing prescriptions for medicines, products, or services.

Script mills: A prescriber writes prescriptions for drugs that are not medically necessary, often in mass quantities, and often for patients that are not theirs. A script mill scheme may include an illegal remuneration scheme.

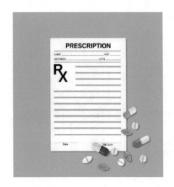

Prescription pad abuse: A prescriber's DEA number or prescription pad is stolen, and is used to write prescriptions to be sold on the black market.

Providing false information: A prescriber falsifies information that is inconsistent with the medical record submitted through a prior authorization or other mechanism to justify coverage. For example, the prescriber misrepresents the dates, descriptions of prescriptions or other services provided, or the identity of the individual who provides the services.

Billing-related scenarios

False claims: A provider submits a claim for items or services that were not provided to a patient.

Unreasonable claims: A provider submits claims for equipment, supplies, or services that are not reasonable or necessary for care.

Double billing: A provider submits a claim to a federal program and to either a private insurance company or the patient for the same treatment to receive duplicate payment; or, two different providers submit a claim for the same patient and same procedure, so that both get paid.

Billing for non-covered services: A provider submits a claim for services that are not allowed through the federal program, or knowingly misuses a provider ID or PIN that results in improper billing.

Unbundling services: A provider uses two or more Current Procedural Terminology (CPT) billing codes instead of a single inclusive code on a claim; or, a provider submits multiple bills in an attempt to increase reimbursement for services that were performed within a specified time period and should have been submitted as a single bundled claim.

Failure to code with modifiers: A provider leaves out coding modifiers that align patient documentation with coding. The provider may do this in an attempt to increase claim amounts or qualify for coverage.

Altering medical records: A provider makes changes to a patient's medical record in order to increase claim amount, or to correct incorrect or incomplete records after receiving an audit request.

Compensation programs that incentivize services ordered and revenue generated: A provider creates a program to reward healthcare professionals who generate more business and income for the enterprise, which results in billing the federal government for unnecessary services.

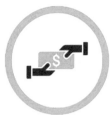

Inappropriate use of place-of-service codes: A provider incorrectly codes the location where a service was provided to take advantage of Medicare's policy to reimburse providers at a higher rate for services provided in their offices and other non-facility locations.

Routine waivers of deductibles and coinsurance: A provider routinely waives patients' cost-sharing amounts as a favor to the patient, professional courtesy, employee benefit, or marketing strategy. The Office of the Inspector General has found that this practice misrepresents the provider's costs, and encourages unnecessary visits and services.

Clustering: A provider uses only one or two middle levels of service codes, in the belief that the charges will eventually average out. The practice leads to some patients being overcharged for services, and others being undercharged.

Upcoding the level of service provided: A provider uses a code for a more expensive service than the one actually provided in order to submit a higher claim for reimbursement.

1.2   Fraud and Abuse Laws; Federal Enforcement Agencies

1.2.1 Major federal fraud and abuse laws

There are five major federal fraud and abuse laws that apply to healthcare providers. As a healthcare professional, it is critical that you know and understand these laws; breaking them could lead to criminal penalties, civil fines, exclusion from federal healthcare programs, and the loss of a medical license.

1.2.1.1 The Federal Anti-Kickback Statute (AKS)

The AKS prohibits providers from intentionally offering, soliciting, or receiving anything of value to generate referrals for items or services payable by any federal health program. What does this mean?

It means that it is a crime to pay for or get paid for referrals that are covered by federal healthcare programs like Medicaid and Medicare.

For example, say a provider receives cash or is offered below-fair-market-value rent on medical offices in exchange for referrals to another provider. That cash, or the difference in monthly rent, is considered a kickback. Both providers—the one offering and the one receiving the kickback—may be found guilty of violating the AKS.

The AKS is a broad statute, and healthcare professionals are often surprised by the range of activities that may be considered a violation of the law, from sports tickets to providing everyday services and amenities.

Providers who are found guilty of violating the AKS could face civil penalties of up to three times the amount of the kickback and criminal penalties that include fines, imprisonment, or both.

1.2.1.2 The Stark Law

The Stark Law, also known as the Physician Self-Referral Law, regulates self-referrals made by physicians. Named for U.S. Congressman Pete Stark, the law is intended to remove potential conflicts of interest, prevent the overuse of services that can drive up costs, and also prevent a captive referral service, which can limit competition.

The Stark Law is a strict liability statute—there does not need to be proof of intent to find that a provider has violated the law.

Under the law, a physician cannot refer a Medicare or Medicaid patient for certain health services to an entity where there is a "financial relationship" with the physician or a member of his or her immediate family. The law defines financial relationship by compensation agreements and ownership or investment interest.

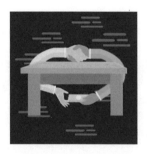

The Stark Law contains several exceptions, including physician services, in-office ancillary services, ownership in publicly traded securities and mutual funds, office space and equipment rental, and a bona fide employment relationship.

Physicians who violate the Stark Law face fines, repayment of claims, and potential exclusion from participation in all Federal healthcare programs.

1.2.1.3 The False Claims Act (FCA)

Designed to protect the government from being overcharged, the FCA prohibits healthcare organizations from "knowingly" making a false record or filing a false claim to a federal healthcare program. Knowingly includes having actual knowledge that a claim is false or acting with "reckless disregard" as to whether a claim is false.

That means that under the FCA, it is a crime to submit claims for payment to Medicare or Medicaid that you know—or should know—are false or fraudulent. For instance, physician who submits claims to Medicare for a higher level of medical services than actually provided or that has included on the patient's medical record can be found guilty of violating the FCA.

Physicians have gone to prison for submitting false healthcare claims.

FCA penalties doubled in August 2016 to between $10,781.40 and $21,562.80 per claim, plus three times the amount of damages that the federal government sustains because of the false claim. Criminal penalties for submitting false claims include imprisonment and criminal fines.

1.2.1.4 The Exclusion Statute

The Exclusion Statute is a section of the Social Security Act that explains why healthcare practitioners and entities can be banned from participating in federal healthcare programs. It excludes practitioners who have been convicted of crimes related to Medicare and Medicaid.

An exclusion is a penalty imposed on a provider. A provider who has been excluded is prohibited from collecting payment from a federal healthcare program for the duration of the exclusion period.

According to the Exclusion Statute, the OIG must exclude providers and suppliers from participation in all federal healthcare programs if they have been convicted of the following violations:

Excluded providers are not automatically reinstated once the exclusion period is over. The provider has to apply for reinstatement and receive authorized notice from the OIG that reinstatement has been granted.

- Medicare fraud

- Patient abuse or neglect

- Felony convictions related to fraud, theft, embezzlement, breach of fiduciary responsibility, or other financial misconduct in connection with the delivery of a healthcare item or service

- Felony convictions for unlawful manufacture, distribution, prescription, or dispensing of controlled substances

There are two types of exclusions:

- **Mandatory exclusions.** The OIG is required to exclude providers found guilty of felonies and criminal offenses such as Medicare and Medicaid fraud for a minimum of five years.

- **Permissive exclusions.** The OIG has discretionary authority to decide whether to exclude providers found guilty of other offenses, such as losing a state license to practice, failing to repay student loans, conviction of certain misdemeanors, or failing to provide quality care.

 It is the responsibility of the employer to routinely check the List of Excluded Individuals and Entities (LEIE) to ensure that new hires and current employees are not on the list. You can access the OIG Exclusions Database online at https://exclusions.oig.hhs.gov. The OIG updates the database each month.

1.2.1.5 The Civil Monetary Penalties Law (CMPL)

The Civil Monetary Penalties Law (CMPL) authorizes the OIG to impose civil monetary penalties (CMPs), assessments, and program exclusions against any person found guilty of submitting false or fraudulent claims for Medicare or Medicaid payment. Penalties vary according to the type of violation.

Federal agencies impose penalties according to the Federal Sentencing Guidelines. In the culpability scoring set out in the guidelines, there are four mitigating factors that can result in reduced penalties and fines:

- Whether or not the organization had an effective compliance program

- Whether or not a violation was reported promptly

- Whether or not the organization cooperated with the government investigators

- Whether or not the organization accepted responsibility for the violation "culpability score"

1.2.2 Federal enforcement agencies

A number of federal agencies are involved in enforcing the fraud and abuse laws discussed above. Although each agency has a different role, they collaborate to address fraudulent and abusive practices in federal healthcare programs.

1.2.2.1 Office of the Inspector General, Department of Health and Human Services (OIG)

The OIG's mission is to fight waste, fraud and abuse in Medicare, Medicaid and more than 100 other HHS programs. The agency employs a national network of audits, investigations and inspections to combat fraud, waste, and abuse and improve the efficiency of the HHS programs.

1.2.2.2 Centers for Medicaid and Medicare Services (CMS)

The CMS is the federal agency within the U.S. Department of Health and Human Services (HHS) that administers the Medicare, Medicaid, SCHIP, Health Insurance Portability and Accountability Act of 1996 (HIPAA), Clinical Laboratory Improvement Amendments (CLIA), and other health-related programs. The agency is tasked with preventing, detecting, and investigating potential Medicare fraud and abuse.

The CMS has stepped up efforts to prevent fraud by increasing provider and supplier enrollment screening. The screening program focuses on increasing the number of site visits to Medicare-enrolled providers and suppliers; enhancing address verification software to improve detection of vacant or invalid addresses or commercial mail receiving agencies (CMRAs); deactivating providers and suppliers that have not billed Medicare in the last 13 months; and monitoring and identifying potentially invalid addresses on a monthly basis through additional data analysis by checking against the U.S. Postal Service address verification database.

1.2.2.3 Department of Justice (DOJ)

The Department of Justice is the federal agency responsible for enforcing the laws of the country; providing federal leadership in preventing and controlling crime; seeking punishment for those found guilty of breaking the law; and ensuring fair and impartial administration of justice.

The DOJ collaborates with the HHS to coordinate federal, state, and local law enforcement activities to address healthcare fraud and abuse under the Healthcare Fraud and Abuse Control Program (HCFAC).

The DOJ Yates Memo: Personal accountability for company violations

In 2015, the Department of Justice released the "Yates Memo," a policy memorandum titled "Individual Accountability for Corporate Wrongdoing." The memo signaled the DOJ's policy shift to focusing investigative efforts on **individual** wrongdoers within a corporation.

Under the new policy, the DOJ is pressuring providers under investigation for violations of the False Claims Act, Stark Law, and/or Anti-Kickback Statute to present evidence of individual wrongdoing.

This means that decision-makers may be held personally liable for healthcare fraud violations at their companies.

This was the case for a healthcare company in Columbia, South Carolina, which was fined $237.4 million in 2015 for Stark Law violations after the DOJ found that the company had entered into sweetheart deals with physicians. The physicians referred outpatient procedures to the company in exchange for compensation that far exceeded fair market value, and included money received from Medicare for the referred procedures.

The DOJ also pursued individual action against the company's CEO for the violations. In 2016, the DOJ reached a settlement with the CEO for $1 million dollars and a 4-year ban from federal healthcare programs.

In November 2018, Deputy Attorney General Rod Rosenstein delivered a speech announcing changes to the Yates Memo. While the new policy revisions still reflect a continued focus on individual accountability, the revisions ease the burden for awarding cooperation credit to corporations that meaningfully assist a government investigation and provide more flexibility to DOJ attorneys in resolving these matters.

1.2.2.4 Medicaid Fraud Control Units (MFCUs)

MFCUs operate in every state to investigate and prosecute Medicaid provider fraud, as well as patient abuse or neglect in healthcare facilities and board and care facilities. The units typically operate out of the state's Attorney General's office and employ teams of investigators, attorneys, and auditors.

1.2.2.5 Healthcare Fraud Prevention and Enforcement Action Team (HEAT)

HEAT is a joint initiative of the DOJ and HHS formed in 2009 to raise the priority of Medicare fraud enforcement.

HEAT efforts include the creation of interagency task force teams to fight fraud and abuse, as well as the launch of the Stop Medicare Fraud website (https://www.stopmedicarefraud.gov/index.html), which provides information about how to identify, prevent and report Medicare fraud.

1.3 The 7 Components of an Effective Compliance Program

A comprehensive compliance program is an essential tool for healthcare organizations to help them comply with federal and state laws and to provide them with the framework to detect, deter and prevent fraud and abusive practices. An effective program may have the added benefit of speeding up and optimizing claim payments, minimizing billing errors and reducing the chance of an audit.

The Patient Protection and Affordable Care Act imposed mandatory compliance programs for all Medicare and Medicaid providers. It also required the HHS to circulate "core elements" and set an effective date for compliance programs.

The Office of the Inspector General recommends a seven-component compliance program that can provide a solid basis for a voluntary compliance program. This section considers each of the seven components in detail.

How to develop an effective compliance program

1. **Conduct internal monitoring and auditing**
2. **Implement compliance and practice standards**
3. **Designate a compliance officer or contact**
4. **Conduct appropriate training and education**
5. **Respond appropriately to detected offenses and take corrective action**
6. **Develop open lines of communication with employees**
7. **Enforce disciplinary standards through well-publicized guidelines**

1.3.1 Component 1: Conduct internal monitoring and auditing

Don't wait for a federal agency to come in and audit your company. Stay on top of compliance through regular monitoring and internal auditing activities.

OIG guidance states that ongoing evaluation of your practice is critical to avoid wrongdoing and to correct problems in a timely manner. Likewise, audits conducted on a regular basis can help identify risk areas that can drive policy changes or address misconduct.

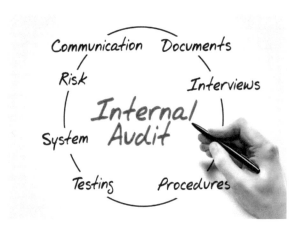

In-house chart audits are your practice's best defense against coding/billing irregularities that may become apparent in a third-party audit. In addition, internal audits tell government enforcement agents that your organization is committed to proactively addressing concerns, and can help support your position that there any alleged fraudulent practices were unintentional.

Internal audits may have the added benefit of increasing revenue through the detection of uncaptured or miscoded services.

1.3.2 Component 2: Implement compliance and practice standards

An effective compliance program establishes a best-practices policy and implementation process for proper decision-making regarding compliance issues. The policy includes all levels of employees, vendors and outside contractors, and clearly states consequences associated with non-compliance.

The policy and procedures should be developed by looking at areas of risk. They should reflect a company-wide code of conduct that stems from the company's mission, vision and values and should address areas of risk.

Procedures should include a periodic review of the policy and procedures to ensure that it is being followed.

 Remember! the only thing worse than not having a policy in place is having a policy in place and not following it.

1.3.3 Component 3: Designate a compliance officer or contact

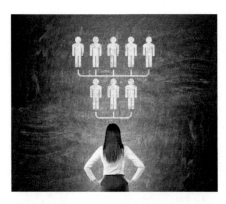

The role of the compliance officer is critical to the success of your program. This person is tasked with implementing and monitoring the compliance program, and revising it whenever necessary.

The compliance officer will report compliance activities and concerns to the governing body, coordinate education and training, and conduct screenings to make sure no current employees are on the OIG Exclusions List and to avoid hiring employees on the Exclusions List.

Here are some things to consider when appointing a compliance officer:

- The compliance officer should be a **strong leader** with an **independent** and effective personality
- The Compliance Officer should be **separate from the legal and finance departments** to ensure that reviews are independent and objective
- The compliance officer should be appointed as a **high-level employee** with adequate resources and authority to effectively implement the compliance program

1.3.4 Component 4: Conduct appropriate training and education

Staff education is the first line of defense when implementing and enforcing an effective compliance program. A strong education and training program makes employees aware of risk and articulates their roles for keeping the company in compliance.

New employees should receive training at the time they are hired and all employees should receive annual refresher courses on core topics. (The CMS requires all Fraud, Waste and Abuse training to be completed within 90 days of hiring and annually thereafter).

Here are some key items to consider when developing a training program:

- Pay close attention to high-risk areas for specialized staff
- Maintain a training log and calendar, and provide ample notice of all training events
- Keep detailed documentation and attestation of employee training

1.3.5 Component 5: Respond appropriately to detected offenses and take corrective action

What should you do if you discover a potential act of fraud, waste, or abuse? First, remember what you should **never** do: **Never** try to cover up the problem. Don't ignore it, and don't alter records. Instead, take action immediately: Stop or modify the alleged misconduct immediately, and document any internal investigation conducted.

Detected offenses that require an immediate response may include the following:

- An allegation of a violation of law
- A report of improper conduct
- A potential government overpayment
- A potential overpayment by a third-party payer
- The possibility of whistleblower activity

Here are key items to document during your internal investigation:

- The report of the alleged misconduct
- A detailed account of the investigation process
- A list of documents reviewed
- A list of all employees interviewed
- Notes and additional documents from the interviews

- A description of changes made to policy/procedures as a result of the investigation
- Disciplinary actions taken as a result of the investigation

This documentation would be a part of your final report for the investigation, and would be used to decide on any remedial actions taken.

In the event of alleged misconduct, you may also decide to discuss the matter with your attorney to determine whether you should exercise attorney-client privilege.

1.3.6 Component 6: Develop open lines of communication with employees

As with education and training, keeping the lines of communication open with company employees can significantly strengthen a compliance program and help a company address and manage problems early and effectively.

Employees should be urged to share any compliance concerns they have as soon as they become aware of them. Prompt disclosure allows the company to catch and remedy or self-disclose problems early on, instead of getting tangled up in a whistleblower case.

Employees need to know that they do not have to fear retaliation for reporting a compliance issue, and they should be provided with multiple methods of reporting to help expedite the communication.

Acceptable methods for reporting compliance concerns include:

- A compliance hotline
- An email address
- A Drop Box account
- In-person communication

Best practices suggest that reporting methods include an anonymous hotline. Why? Because an anonymous hotline serves as a safety valve and an early warning system that can give a company a heads-up in time to remedy the situation. Despite assurances that they will not suffer retaliation for reporting concerns, many employees still worry their jobs will affected if they report an issue. According to an Ernst and Young survey conducted in 2002, one in five workers had knowledge of workplace fraud, and 39 percent were more likely to report it if they were given an anonymous option. Moreover, nearly half of all hotline calls were made outside of business hours.

Employees who do not feel they can safely report an issue may choose to become a "whistleblowers." Under the False Claims Act, a whistleblower is someone who reports evidence of fraud against federal programs to a government enforcement agency. The FCA protects whistleblowers from harassment, discrimination, suspension, and termination from their employers. A whistleblower who is an original source of information, known as a Qui Tam Relator, can sue the company for violations of the FCA and receive between 15 and 30 percent of money recovered by the government, whether that money is obtained through a judgment or a settlement.

The potential for whistleblower activity is another reason for a company to promptly follow up on reports of misconduct and carefully document any investigation using a log and report form.

1.3.7 Component 7: Enforce disciplinary standards through well-publicized guidelines

Employees should have a clear understanding of the consequences they face for compliance misconduct. This can be accomplished by developing well-defined guidelines and making sure that employees have access to them.

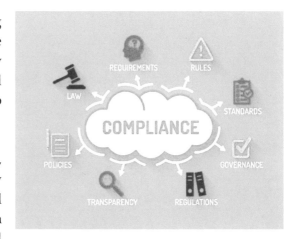

Disciplinary standards must be fair, commensurate with the offense, consistently applied, and clearly communicated to all employees. Employees should receive a written version of the policy, and it should be included in training sessions. Employees should understand the remedial disciplinary steps that can lead to termination.

The Office of the Inspector General recommends five points to Include in a disciplinary policy:

- Language that clearly states that noncompliance will be punished
- Language that clearly states that failure to report noncompliance will be punished
- An outline of disciplinary procedures
- A list of the parties responsible for appropriate disciplinary action
- Language that promises discipline will be fair and consistent

1.3.8 The costs and consequences of a reactive compliance policy

Taking a reactive rather than proactive approach to compliance can be costly, as discussed in this "True Cost of Compliance" benchmark study conducted by Ponemon Institute.

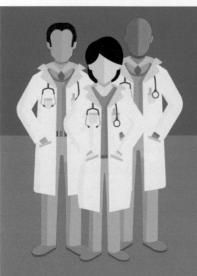

Healthcare Compliance:
Costs vs Benefits

Within the healthcare industry, the focus has increasingly turned toward compliance, and there are multiple regulations that prompt the need for implementation of an effective program.

COSTS of Being Reactive

BENEFITS of Being Proactive

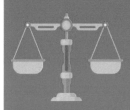

It's the law, so criminal charges come into play. Enforcement has been increased over the last several years.

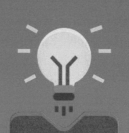

Staff confidence and morale will benefit from extra training and knowledge. "Knowledge is power" is especially applicable in any medical setting.

Reputation matters more than ever. News travels fast and a physician's reputation has a direct impact on the success of the practice.

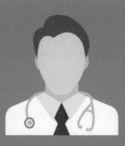

Showing that you've committed time and resources to compliance shows the community and your staff that you believe in doing things the right way.

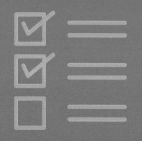

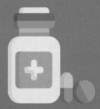

Patient outcomes may be affected by lack of safety.

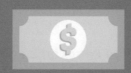

Having a full compliance program in place leads to better communication and uncovering potential problems.

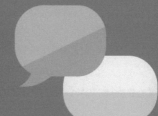

The impact may be monetary via fines and penalties.

Comprehensive Healthcare Compliance Management Solutions

CONFIDENCE INCLUDED

Creating confidence among compliance professionals through education, resources, and support

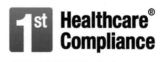

1st Healthcare® Compliance

888.54.FIRST 1sthcc.com

(http://www.ponemon.org/local/upload/file/True_Cost_of_Compliance_Report_copy.pdf)
Possible costs include:

- **Legal consequences:** It's the law, so criminal charges come into play. Enforcement has been increased over the last several years, and the news is full of violation cases. See the enforcement actions section of the OIG website for recent examples. (https://oig.hhs.gov/fraud/enforcement/state/index.asp)

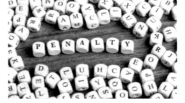

- **Reputation:** News travels fast in the digital world, and a physician's reputation has a direct impact on the success of the practice. Most patients check provider reviews online.

- **Patient outcomes:** Patient health may be at risk by noncompliant practices, such as neglecting to follow staph prevention rules (https://www.yahoo.com/beauty/only-1-in-5-nurses-follow-the-right-safety-150255556.html).

- **Financial impact**: In addition to paying monetary fines and penalties for healthcare violations, a provider's practice may also lose business as peers and patients learn about the situation.

What did you learn? Discussion topics for Chapter 1

➢ What constitutes fraud in a healthcare setting? What are some examples of healthcare fraud?

➢ What constitutes waste in a healthcare setting? What are some examples of healthcare waste?

➢ What constitutes abuse in a healthcare setting? What are some examples of healthcare abuse?

➢ What are the five federal laws that address fraud, waste and abuse in healthcare?

➢ What are the criminal and civil consequences of fraud, waste and abuse violations? How can these consequences impact a healthcare provider's business?

➢ What are the seven components of an effective compliance program to prevent fraud, waste and abuse? What are the consequences of relying on a "reactive" compliance policy?

Online Resources

"Adjustments to Civil Monetary Penalty Amounts." The 2015 Federal Civil Penalties Inflation Adjustment Act requires all agencies to annually adjust for inflation the civil monetary penalties that can be imposed under the statutes administered by the agency. This final rule from the SEC performs the first annual adjustment for inflation of the maximum amount of civil monetary penalties. https://www.sec.gov/rules/final/2017/33-10276.pdf

"Comparison of the Anti-Kickback Statute and Stark Law." This HEAT chart compares the laws. https://oig.hhs.gov/compliance/provider-compliance-training/files/starkandakscharthandout508.pdf

"Compliance Program Guidance for Hospitals." An excerpt from the Federal Register/Vol. 53 No. 35 2/23/1998 with guidance to assist hospitals develop effective internal controls that promote adherence to Federal and State law. https://oig.hhs.gov/authorities/docs/cpghosp.pdf

"Criteria for implementing section 1128(b)(7) exclusion authority April 18, 2016." A revised policy statement from the OIG regarding exclusions imposed for fraud, waste and abuse violations. https://oig.hhs.gov/exclusions/files/1128b7exclusion-criteria.pdf

"Healthcare Compliance Program Tips." An outline of the seven elements of an effective compliance program.https://www.crimcheck.com/wp-content/uploads/2013/03/Health-Care-Compliance-Program-Tips.pdf

"Healthcare Programs: Fraud and Abuse; Revisions to the Office of Inspector General's Exclusion Authorities—Final rule." This final rule amends the regulations relating to exclusion authorities under the authority of the OIG. https://www.gpo.gov/fdsys/pkg/FR-2017-01-12/pdf/2016-31390.pdf

"Laws Against Healthcare Fraud Resource Guide." A 6-page CMS e-publication that provides an overview of some of the major federal fraud and abuse laws. https://www.cms.gov/Medicare-Medicaid-Coordination/Fraud-Prevention/Medicaid-Integrity-Education/Downloads/fwa-laws-resourceguide.pdf

"Medicare Fraud & Abuse: Prevention, Detection and Reporting." A 20-page CMS e-publication that explores fraud and abuse issues related to Medicare. https://www.cms.gov/Outreach-and-Education/Medicare-Learning-Network-MLN/MLNProducts/downloads/Fraud_and_Abuse.pdf

"OIG Compliance Program for Individual and Small Group Physician Practices." This Federal Register Notice sets forth the issued Compliance Program Guidance for Individual and Small Group Physician Practices developed by the OIG. https://oig.hhs.gov/authorities/docs/physician.pdf

"Special Advisory Bulletin on the Effect of Exclusion from Participation in Federal Healthcare Programs." This OIG bulletin describes the scope and effect of the legal prohibition on payment by Federal healthcare programs for items or services furnished (1) by an excluded person or (2) at the medical direction or on the prescription of an excluded person. https://oig.hhs.gov/exclusions/files/sab-05092013.pdf

Chapter 2

HIPAA

Overview

In this chapter, you will learn how the HIPAA Privacy, Security and Enforcement Rules impact healthcare providers, the key components of a HIPAA compliance plan, and the consequences of HIPAA noncompliance.

Chapter Outline

2.1   The HIPAA Privacy Rule
2.2   Entities addressed by HIPAA
2.3   Personal health representatives
2.4   Protected health information (PHI)
2.5   Uses and disclosures of PHI
2.6   Minimum necessary standard
2.7   Notice of privacy practices
2.8   The Rights of the Individual Under the HIPAA Privacy Rule
2.9   Privacy Rule Administrative Requirements
2.10   The HIPAA Security Rule
2.11   Reporting Non-Compliance
2.12   Breach Notification Rule
2.13   The HIPAA Enforcement Rule

Learning Objectives

After completing this chapter, you should be able to do the following:

✓ Understand how the HIPAA Privacy Rule has evolved, the entities it covers and the information it protects.

✓ Describe the elements of an effective HIPAA compliance plan.

✓ Understand the Standards and Implementation Specifications of the HIPAA Security Rule, and how HITECH and the Omnibus Final Rule have impacted the Security Rule.

✓ Explain the components of an effective breach notification policy.

✓ Explain how HIPAA rules are enforced, including civil monetary penalties and individual liability.

2.1   The HIPAA Privacy Rule

Physicians have long recognized the critical importance of protecting a patient's privacy. In addition to moral and ethical considerations, patient confidentiality is essential to achieving positive health outcomes. If patients are concerned that their medical details could become public knowledge, they might be reluctant to share health information, fearing that it might damage their reputation, put their job at risk or put them in danger. Patients and caregivers

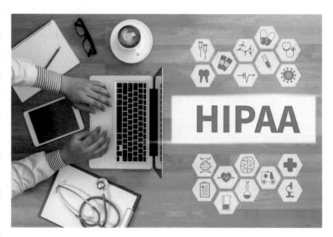

need a relationship built on trust and confidentiality if the care is to be effective.

The HIPAA Privacy Rule was designed to address this critical patient care issue—especially in light of the increased use of electronic storage and transfer of records. The Rule, the first comprehensive federal protection of the privacy of health information, created national standards to protect individuals' medical records and other personal health information (PHI).

The Privacy Rule requires certain healthcare providers to implement safeguards that protect the privacy of PHI, and regulates the ways that the providers can use and disclose PHI without a patient's authorization. The Rule also provides patients with rights over their health information, such as the right to examine their health records, to obtain a copy of them, and to request corrections.

The Privacy Rule was designed to do the following:

• It gives patients more control over their health information.

• It sets boundaries on the use and release of health records.

- It establishes safeguards that healthcare providers and others must implement to protect the privacy of health information.

- It holds violators accountable, with civil and criminal penalties that can be imposed for violating patients' privacy rights.

- It seeks to strike a balance when there is a public need for disclosure of some forms of data—for example, to protect public health.

The Privacy Rule also gives patients the ability to make informed choices when seeking care, and reimbursement for care, based on how their PHI may be used:

- It enables patients to find out how their PHI may be used, and to ask about certain PHI disclosures that have been made.

- It limits the release of information to the minimum necessary needed to achieve the intended purpose.

- It gives patients the right to examine and obtain a copy of their own health records and to request corrections.

- It empowers individuals to control certain uses and disclosures of their PHI.

2.2   Entities Addressed by HIPAA

The Privacy Rule establishes which entity types must comply with the HIPAA regulations, and it provides compliance guidelines.

HIPAA applies to covered entities (CEs), which include healthcare providers that perform standard electronic transactions, health plans, and healthcare clearinghouses. Third parties, known as business associates (BAs), that have access to patient information must also comply with HIPAA.

2.2.1 Covered entities

These are the entities that are required to comply with HIPAA rules:

- **Health plan:** With certain exceptions, a health plan is an individual or group plan that pays for medical care. The law specifically includes many types of organizations and government programs as health plans, such as insurance companies (individual or group), Medicare, Medicaid, Children's Health Insurance Program (CHIP), Civilian Health and Medical Program of the Uniformed Services (CHAMPUS), and prescription drug plans.

- **Healthcare clearinghouse:** A clearinghouse is a public or private entity—including a billing service, repricing company, community health management information system or community health information system and "value-added" networks and switches—that acts as a go-between for CEs (for example a healthcare provider and insurance company) to provide the following services:

- o Process or facilitate the processing of health information received from another entity in a nonstandard format or containing nonstandard data content into standard data elements or a standard transaction.

- o Receive a standard transaction from another entity to process or facilitate the processing of health information into nonstandard format or nonstandard data content for the receiving entity.

For example: A healthcare claims clearinghouse would review an insurance claim for errors before submitting it to the payer, and then notify the healthcare provider that the claim has been accepted or denied.

- **Healthcare provider:** These are individuals, organizations or entities that provide, bill, or are paid for medical or health services as part of their business. Examples include doctors, nurses, dentists, psychologists, nursing homes, hospitals, and pharmacies. Healthcare refers to care, services, or supplies related to the health of an individual, including preventive, diagnostic, therapeutic, rehabilitative, maintenance, or palliative care, and counseling, service, assessment, or procedures with respect to the physical or mental condition, or functional status, of an individual; and the sale or dispensing of a drug, device, equipment, or other item requiring a prescription.

- **Affiliated covered entity:** Affiliated CEs are legally separate entities that are affiliated with a CE under common ownership. An example is an integrated delivery network that includes hospitals, medical groups, and long-term care facilities.

- **Organized healthcare arrangement:** There are certain operational arrangements among entities that require the participants to share PHI. An example would be doctors who are affiliated with a university faculty and treat patients in a hospital or health system. For the purposes of HIPAA, a key factor of determining whether an organized healthcare arrangement is a CE is if the patient is aware of the arrangement.

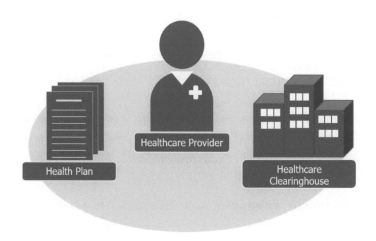

2.2.2 Business associates

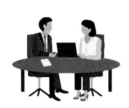

A CE's BAs must also comply with HIPAA requirements. A BA is a person or an entity that is not part of the CE's workforce but performs activities on behalf of the CE that involve the use or disclosure of PHI.

The types of functions or activities for which a person or entity may be considered a BA include payment or healthcare operations activities, as well as many other functions or activities regulated by the Administrative Simplification Rules, such as legal, actuarial, accounting, consulting, data aggregation, management, administrative, accreditation, and financial services. Such activities include:

- Claims processing or administration
- Data analysis, processing, or administration
- Utilization review
- Quality assurance
- Billing
- Benefits management
- Practice management
- Repricing

Examples of BAs include:

- A third-party administrator that assists with claims processing.
- A CPA firm whose accounting services to a healthcare provider involve access to PHI.
- An attorney whose legal services to a health plan involve access to PHI.
- A consultant who performs utilization reviews for a hospital.
- A healthcare clearinghouse that translates a claim from a non-standard format into a standard transaction on behalf of a healthcare provider, and forwards the processed transaction to a payer.
- An independent medical transcriptionist who provides transcription services to a physician.
- A pharmacy benefits manager who manages a health plan's pharmacist network.

Once a CE determines that an entity or an individual with which it has a business relationship meets the definition of a BA, the CE is responsible for ensuring that the third party complies with HIPAA. This is done with a contract or other agreement between the CE and BA. The

Who are your Business Associates?

Definition of a Business Associate

A Business Associate is a person or entity that performs certain functions or activities that involve the use or disclosure of protected health information on behalf of, or provides services to, a covered entity.

Examples

A third party <u>administrator</u> that assists a health plan with claims processing

An independent medical <u>transcriptionist</u> that provides transcription services to a physician

A <u>CPA firm</u> whose accounting services to a health care provider involve access to protected health information

An <u>attorney</u> whose legal services to a health plan involve access to protected health information

Do I need a Business Associate Agreement for the phone company or the internet provider? They could access my patient information, so we need a BAA with them, right?

BAAs are not necessary with certain organizations considered to be mere conduits. Examples are the U.S. Postal Service, some private couriers, telephone companies, and Internet Service Providers. This is because a conduit transports the information, but does not access it. No disclosure is intended by the covered entity (healthcare provider) and there is low likelihood of disclosure of PHI in these situations.

What about the landlord or the cleaning service? They have access to the office where we keep PHI.

It is unnecessary to have a BAA with the cleaning service because they are not contracted to perform services involving use or disclosure of PHI. However, you need to have reasonable safeguards in place to protect PHI. Ideally, you should store paper PHI in a locked cabinet.

Do I need to have a BAA with my accountant? She's been working with us for years, but isn't an employee.

It is common to overlook a business associate who has been working with your organization for a long period of time. However, if an independent contractor is providing services such as accounting or anything that involves PHI, then you must have a BAA in place.

Comprehensive Healthcare Compliance Management Solutions

CONFIDENCE INCLUDED

Creating confidence among compliance professionals through education, resources, and support

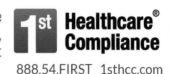

888.54.FIRST 1sthcc.com

contract, known as a business associate agreement (BAA), is a written arrangement that specifies each party's responsibilities with regard to PHI.

2.2.2.1 Identifying BAs

Managing the many relationships within a healthcare organization can be a daunting task, and determining which entities qualify as BAs is not always straightforward. It is important to examine each vendor relationship to determine whether a BA relationship exists and requires a written BAA.

There can be serious consequences for not identifying BAs or not formalizing the relationship with a BAA. Consider this case: In 2018, Pagosa Springs Medical Center (PSMC) agreed to pay $111,400 to settle an OCR investigation regarding potential HIPAA violations. The investigation revealed, among other things, that PSMC used Google to maintain its web-based scheduling calendar for patient appointments without signing a BAA with Google before the online company disclosed, stored, and saved PHI.[1]

2.2.2.2 Exceptions to the BA standard

The Privacy Rule does not require CEs to have a BAA in place before PHI can be disclosed in these situations:

- Disclosures by a CE to a healthcare provider for treatment. For example:
  - A hospital does not need a BAA with a specialist to whom it refers a patient and transmits the patient's medical chart for treatment purposes.
  - A doctor does not need a BAA with a lab in order to disclose PHI to treat a patient.
  - A hospital lab does not need a BAA to disclose PHI to a reference laboratory to treat a patient.
- Disclosures by a CE to a health plan sponsor, such as an employer, by a group health plan, or by the health insurance issuer or HMO that provides health insurance benefits or coverage for the group health plan.
- Collecting and sharing PHI by a public benefits program, such as Medicare, and an agency other than the agency administering the health plan, such as the Social Security Administration.

---

[1] https://www.hhs.gov/about/news/2018/12/11/colorado-hospital-failed-to-terminate-former-employees-access-to-electronic-protected-health-information.html

- Disclosures by a healthcare provider to a health plan for payment, or when the healthcare provider accepts a discounted rate to participate in the health plan's network.

- With individuals or organizations whose services do not involve the use or disclosure of PHI and do not have more than incidental access to PHI.

- With a person or organization that is simply a conduit for PHI, such as the US Postal Service, some private couriers, and their electronic equivalents.

- Among CEs that participate in an organized healthcare arrangement (OHCA) to make disclosures that relate to the joint healthcare activities of the OHCA.

- Where a group health plan purchases insurance from a health insurance issuer or an HMO.

- Where a CE purchases a health plan product or other insurance, for example reinsurance, from an insurer.

- For research purposes, either with patient authorization or as a limited data set.

- When a financial institution processes financial transactions for healthcare or health plan premiums payment (unless functions that are above and beyond payment processing activities are performed, such as account receivable functions).

2.2.3 Hybrid entities

A hybrid entity is a single legal entity that performs both covered and non-covered functions, and that designates certain units as healthcare components. A hybrid entity must comply with HIPAA in some regards, but not others. If a CE opts not to hybridize, then it and all of its components are subject to HIPAA.

If a CE does decide to operate as a hybrid entity, it must clearly define and designate the healthcare component(s) that do and do not perform CE and/or BA functions, and document that designation. For example, the research arm of a hybrid entity that functions as a healthcare provider and engages in standard electronic transactions would be subject to the Privacy Rule.

It is the entity's responsibility to decide whether it is a hybrid entity, and which of its components would be considered healthcare services. An entity should therefore carefully review its operations to determine which services and activities come under HIPAA.

---

[2] https://www.hhs.gov/hipaa/for-professionals/compliance-enforcement/agreements/umass/index.html

2.3   Personal Representatives

A patient has the right to designate someone else to participate in their healthcare or to act on their behalf. These designated individuals are known as personal representatives, and have the same rights as the patient with regard to the patient's PHI. For example, a personal representative can request access to the person's PHI, request an accounting of disclosures, and can authorize PHI use or disclosure.

The personal representative may have broad authority to act on the patient's behalf, for example in the case of the parent of a minor or the legal guardian of a mentally incompetent adult, or the authority may be limited. If the personal representative's authority is limited, the CE or BA must make sure it understands and observes the limits set by the patient. For example, if a personal representative is given permission to only authorize a specific treatment, such as artificial life support, the CE cannot ask the personal representative to authorize use or disclosure of the patient's PHI for marketing purposes.

CEs and BAs should consult state law to check whether there are additional regulations regarding the authority of personal representatives. The Privacy Rule defers to state laws that expressly address a parent's right to access their offspring's medical information.

2.3.1 Situations of abuse, neglect, and endangerment

If a CE has reason to believe that an individual is the victim of domestic violence, abuse, or neglect by their personal representative, or believes that sharing medical information about a patient to a personal representative could result in harm to the patient, the CE can choose not to recognize the designated person as the patient's personal representative.

2.4   Protected Health Information

2.4.1 PHI

Under the HIPAA Privacy Rule, PHI is defined as individually identifiable health information (IIHI) held or transmitted by a CE or BA in any form or media, including electronic, paper and oral, that identifies the patient or could reasonably be used to identify the patient, and relates to the following:

- A patient's past, present, or future physical or mental health condition
- All healthcare provided to the patient
- Past, present, or future payments for treatment provided to the patient

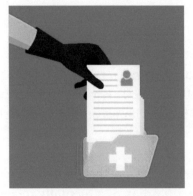

PHI is typically found in medical forms, documents, and communications, such as laboratory reports, radiology reports, and hospital bills.

Types of PHI data include the following 18 identifiers of the individual or of relatives, employers, or household members of the individual if it is associated with health information:

- Name
- Addresses: In particular, anything more specific than the state, including street address, city, county, precinct, and in most cases zip code, and their equivalent geocodes
- Telephone number
- Fax number
- Email address
- Dates (except for year): date of birth, date of death, date of service, date of admittance, date of discharge
- Social security number
- Medical record numbers
- Account numbers
- Health plan beneficiary numbers
- Certification/license numbers
- Vehicle identifiers and serial numbers, including license plate numbers
- Device identifiers and serial numbers
- Internet Protocol (IP) addresses
- Web Universal Resource Locations (URLs)
- Biometric identifier (fingerprint/voiceprint)
- Full-face photographic image
- Other unique identifying numbers, characteristics or codes

Is it PHI?

When you are determining whether patient information should be considered PHI, the relationship of the information with medical circumstances is key. Identifying information alone that is not related to treatment or payment, such as personal names, residential addresses, or phone numbers, would not necessarily be designated as PHI.

In the wrong hands, any of these data types could be used to identify somebody and link them to their private medical information.

2.4.2 Non-PHI

Not all individual identifiable information is considered PHI. For example, a CE's employment records, or student health information in education records that are protected by the Family Educational Rights and Privacy Act (FERPA) are not considered PHI because the information is not linked to health records that could compromise an individual's medical privacy.

In addition, some health information isn't considered PHI because it can't be used to identify an individual, or because it is not created, received, maintained, or transmitted by a CE or BA.

2.4.3 De-identified PHI

De-identified patient data is information that cannot be used to link an individual to healthcare situations. There are no privacy restrictions on de-identified health information, and it is considered a valuable asset to the healthcare community because it can be used to improve care, estimate the costs of care, and support public health initiatives.

De-identified PHI is a medical record that has had all "direct identifiers" such as those listed in Section 2.4.1, to the point where the patient can't be recognized.

There are several accepted methods for de-identifying PHI in order to use it for studies, cost analysis, etc. For example, a qualified statistician could wipe data clean and declare PHI unrecognizable; or, a CE could remove the 18 direct identifiers that constitute PHI data and stipulate that, to the best of its knowledge, the data could not be used alone or in combination with other information to determine a patient's identity.

2.4.4 Psychotherapy notes

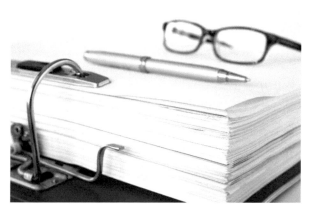

Psychotherapy notes are a subset of PHI that receive special consideration under HIPAA, because they may contain personal notes and sensitive information that is not needed for treatment, payment, or healthcare operations. (See Section 2.5.2.1.2.)

Psychotherapy notes refer to any notes taken by a mental health professional while providing mental health treatment, such as private, group, joint, or family counseling. The notes are kept separate from the rest of the patient's medical record and are not typically disclosed for other purposes.

Under the Privacy Rule, psychotherapy notes are specifically excluded from a patient's general right to access or inspect their own medical records (see Section 2.8.1). Moreover, CEs must get specific authorization from a patient before psychotherapy notes can be disclosed to a third party. The patient's request must be recorded on a form used exclusively to document the authorization to release psychotherapy notes.

Psychotherapy notes do not include PHI kept elsewhere in the medical record, nor the following:

- Medication prescription and monitoring

- Counseling session start and stop times

- Types and frequencies of treatment provided

- Results of clinical tests

- Any summary of the following items: Diagnosis, functional status, treatment plan, symptoms, prognosis, patient progress

2.5 Uses and Disclosures of PHI

HIPAA protects an individual's right to keep PHI private and confidential. However, there are a variety of reasons that healthcare providers need to use and share PHI, such as communicating with insurance companies to expedite payment, or sharing PHI among healthcare providers for patient care. Effectively sharing this information is an essential and critical component of providing healthcare.

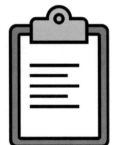

This is a key reason HIPAA exists: In addition to requiring that CEs take measures to keep PHI private and confidential, HIPAA was designed to articulate and regulate the reasons that PHI can be used, shared, or disclosed.

In the broadest sense, PHI can be disclosed for one of two reasons:

1. The patient gives permission.
2. HIPAA allows (or requires) the disclosure.

It's important to understand the difference between the two in order to effectively safeguard and also effectively use and disclose PHI.

2.5.1 The patient gives permission

Patients can give written authorization or consent for use and disclosure of their PHI. Although the words may sound synonymous, there are differences between the two under HIPAA.

2.5.1.1 Consent

CEs need to use and share PHI in order to provide healthcare and receive payment. Individuals expect that their health information will be used as necessary for treatment, billing for that treatment, and, to some extent, to operate the healthcare business. Therefore, the Privacy Rule does not require CEs to obtain a patient's authorization for treatment, payment, and healthcare operations (TPO). CEs may choose to obtain consent for TPO functions, and if so, they can decide how to obtain consent and what to include on a patient consent form.

Patient consent for use and disclosure of PHI for TPO functions cannot be applied to any other uses or disclosures that specifically require written authorization under HIPAA.

2.5.1.2 Authorization

Patient authorization is a detailed document that provides CEs with explicit permission to use and disclose PHI for purposes other than TPO. As a general rule, CEs need to obtain a valid patient authorization before using and disclosing PHI for any reason that is not covered by the required or permitted uses and disclosures under the Privacy Rule. Relying only on a patient's consent, even if they have signed a consent form, when an authorization is required by the Privacy Rule is an unauthorized use of PHI.

A valid authorization must be written in "plain language," meaning that it should be easily read and understood by the CE's patient population, and includes the following information:

- A description of the PHI that the CE plans to use or disclose. The information must be described in a "specific and meaningful fashion."
- The name of the person authorizing the use or disclosure of PHI.
- The name of the person or entity authorized to receive the PHI.
- The purpose of the use or disclosure (the CE can use "at the request of the individual").
- The expiration date of the authorization.
- The authorizing person's signature, and the date the authorization is signed.
- Language that gives the patient the right to revoke the authorization at any time and explains the process for revoking the authorization.
- A statement that the information disclosed may be redisclosed, and may no longer be protected.

- A statement that if the individual does not want to sign the authorization, the CE cannot withhold treatment, payment, enrollment, or eligibility for benefits (unless an exception applies).

2.5.2 HIPAA allows or requires the disclosure

HIPAA allows CEs to use their professional ethics and best judgment to share PHI without obtaining patient authorization in certain situations that are clearly defined by the rule. Six of those situations *allow* the CE to use or disclose the information, and two of those situations *require* the CE to use or disclose the information:

Permitted disclosures:

1. The disclosure is made to the patient.

2. The disclosure is for treatment, payment, or healthcare operations.

3. The patient is given the opportunity to agree or object to the use or disclosure.

4. The use or disclosure is considered incidental.

5. The use or disclosure for public interest or benefit activities.

6. The use or disclosure is a limited data set for research, public health, or healthcare operations.

Required disclosures:

1. A CE is required to disclose PHI if a patient requests access to their PHI, or requests an accounting of disclosures of their PHI (See Section 2.8.5 for patient access).

2. A CE is required to disclose PHI to HHS for the purposes of a compliance investigation, review, or enforcement action. (See Chapter 7 for Enforcement.)

2.5.2.1 Permitted Disclosures

2.5.2.1.1 The disclosure is made to the patient

Under HIPAA, patients have the right to access their information. Therefore, the CE can disclose PHI directly to the patient or the patient's personal representative without an authorization.

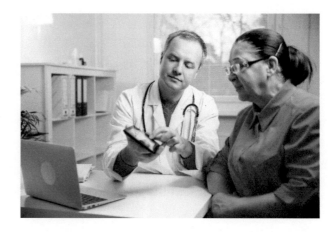

2.5.2.1.2 The disclosure is for treatment, payment, or healthcare operations

A CE is permitted to use and disclose PHI for TPO activities without an authorization. When using or disclosing the PHI for these activities, both the disclosing CE and the receiving CE are required to follow all HIPAA privacy requirements. The disclosing CE is responsible for the PHI right up until the receiving CE has received the information. The disclosing CE is required to use or disclose the PHI in a "permitted and secure" manner, which includes complying with HIPAA Privacy and Security safeguards when sending the PHI, and taking reasonable steps to make sure the PHI is going to the correct address and to the correct person or department.

Once the receiving CE takes possession of the PHI, it is responsible for keeping the PHI private and secure, including with respect to subsequent uses or disclosures, or any breaches that occur.

2.5.2.1.3 Uses and disclosures with an opportunity to agree or object

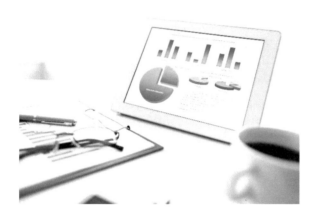

The Privacy Rule permits CEs to use or disclose PHI without obtaining an authorization for certain limited purposes if the individual is given the opportunity to agree or object. These purposes include: using patient information facility directories; using or disclosing PHI for involvement in the individual's care; and, using or disclosing PHI for notification purposes.

The CE can ask the individual for permission, or permission can happen by circumstances that clearly give the individual the opportunity to agree or object. If the individual is incapacitated, in an emergency situation, or not available, CEs generally may use or disclose PHI, if they believe it is in the best interests of the individual.

2.5.2.1.3.1 Facility directories

Some healthcare facilities (for example hospitals) maintain patient directories. CEs are permitted to list certain patient information in these directories, such as names, general condition, religious affiliation, and room numbers. However, the CE must tell the patient about the directory and the information that will be included, and also explain to the patient who will have access to the directory. The patient must be given the chance to restrict the personal information included in the directory, who has access to that information, and to opt out of being included altogether.

The CE can disclose the individual's condition and location to anyone who asks for the individual by name (such as a visitor), and can also disclose religious affiliation to clergy. Clergy do not have to ask for individuals by name when inquiring about patients' religious affiliation.

2.5.2.1.3.2 For notification and other purposes

A CE is permitted to disclose PHI to a patient's family, relatives, or friends, (or even other people that the patient identifies) in these situations:

- The patient gives permission.

- The patient doesn't object.

- The friends or relatives are involved in caring for the patient or paying for treatment.

- The CE uses its professional judgment, believing that disclosing the information is in the patient's best interests, and believes the patient has no objections, for example, if the patient is not present or is unconscious.

For example, a pharmacist can give a filled prescription to a patient's relative, or a surgeon can provide a spouse with information about the procedure while the patient is still unconscious.

Note however, that only information that is relevant to the care at that moment can be shared with others. A caregiver cannot share past medical issues with friends or family if the problems are not directly related to the present issue.

A CE is also permitted to use or disclose PHI to identify, locate, and notify family members or others involved in the patient's care of the individual's location, general condition, or death. PHI can also be disclosed to public or private entities authorized to assist in disaster relief efforts.

2.5.2.1.4 Incidental use and disclosure

The Privacy Rule is not intended to hermetically seal off the flow of medical information. Patients and caregivers depend on the efficient exchange of PHI to manage healthcare and expedite payment.

The Privacy Rule recognizes that this information exchange will occasionally result in "incidental" PHI disclosure, and does not require CEs to eliminate every risk of incidental use or disclosure. In other words, if PHI is used or disclosed as a result of, or as "incident to," an otherwise permitted use or disclosure, it is not considered a violation of the Privacy Rule, so long as the CE has set up reasonable technical and physical safeguards to protect the privacy of the PHI, and the information being shared was limited to the "minimum necessary" (see Section 2.6) as required by the Privacy Rule.

HHS offers these examples of incidental use: A hospital visitor overhears a physician's confidential conversation with another physician; or, a visitor sees patient information on a nursing station whiteboard or on a sign-in sheet.

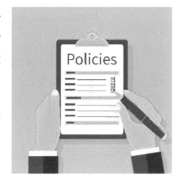

The Rule does **not** permit incidental uses or disclosures if they are the result of a Privacy Rule violation.

2.5.2.1.5 Public interest and benefit activities

CEs are permitted to use and disclose PHI without an individual's authorization for 12 national priority purposes. These disclosures are not required, but the Privacy Rule allows them for public interest. Note that the Rule puts limitations on each purpose to balance the need for individual privacy and the public's need for the information.

The twelve activities are:

1. Disclosures required by law, including by statute, regulation, or court orders.

2. Disclosures supporting public health activities. CEs can disclose to:

   a. Public health authorities in order to prevent or control disease, injury, or disability; and to agencies authorized to receive reports of child abuse and neglect.

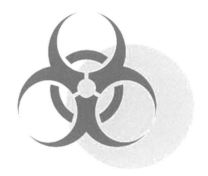

   b. Entities subject to regulation from the Food and Drug Administration (FDA) regarding FDA-regulated products or activities for purposes such as adverse event reporting, tracking of products, product recalls, and post-marketing surveillance.

   c. Individuals who may have contracted or been exposed to a communicable disease (when notification is authorized by law).

   d. Employers, regarding employees (when requested by employers) for information concerning a work-related illness or injury or workplace-related medical surveillance, when the information is needed to comply with the Occupational Safety and Health Administration (OSHA), the Mine Safety and Health Administration (MHSA), or a similar state law.

3. Disclosures to government authorities related to abuse, neglect, or domestic violence.

4. Disclosures for health oversight activities such as audits and investigations necessary for oversight of the healthcare system and government benefit programs.

5. Disclosures for judicial and administrative proceedings if CE receives a PHI request through a court order, administrative tribunal, in response to a subpoena or other

lawful process. In some circumstances, the CE may require assurances that a notice to the individual or a protective order will be provided.

6. Disclosures for law enforcement purposes. The Rule identifies six circumstances where a CE can disclose PHI, subject to specified conditions:

   a. As required by law (including court orders, court-ordered warrants, subpoenas) and administrative requests;

   b. To identify or locate a suspect, fugitive, material witness, or missing person;

   c. In response to a law enforcement official's request for information about a victim or suspected victim of a crime;

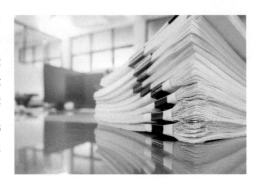

   d. To alert law enforcement of a person's death, if the CE believes that the death is the result of criminal activity;

   e. When a CE believes PHI is evidence of a crime that occurred on its premises; or,

   f. To inform law enforcement about a crime, its victims, or a perpetrator in a medical emergency not occurring on its premises.

7. Disclosures for activities related to a death, including providing PHI to funeral directors, and to coroners or medical examiners to identify a deceased person, determine the cause of death, and perform other functions authorized by law.

8. Disclosures to facilitate organ, eye, or tissue donation from a cadaver.

9. Disclosures for research. A CE can use and disclose PHI for research purposes if it obtains:

   a. Documentation that an alteration or waiver of individuals' authorization for the use or disclosure of PHI for research purposes has been approved by an Institutional Review Board or Privacy Board;

   b. Assurances from the researcher that the PHI will only be used to prepare a research protocol, that the researcher will not remove any PHI from the CE, and that the PHI is essential for the research; or,

   c. Assurances from the researcher that only the PHI of deceased individuals will be used, that the PHI is necessary for the research, and, at the request of the CE, documentation of the death of the individuals about whom information is sought.

10. Disclosures related to serious threats to health or safety, to prevent or lessen a serious and imminent threat to a person or the public. A CE may also disclose PHI to law enforcement if the information is needed to identify or apprehend an escapee or violent criminal.

11. Disclosures that are essential to government functions, such as a military mission, conducting intelligence and national security activities authorized by law, protecting the President, making medical suitability determinations for U.S. State Department employees, protecting the health and safety of inmates or employees in a prison, and determining eligibility for or conducting enrollment in certain government benefit programs.

12. Disclosures related to workers' compensation.

2.5.2.1.6 Limited data set for the purposes of research, public health or healthcare operations

A limited data set is partially de-identified PHI that can be used for research, healthcare operations, and public health purposes, so long as the recipient of the PHI enters into a data use agreement promising specified safeguards for the PHI within the limited data set.

2.5.2.2 Required Disclosures

A CE is required to disclose PHI if a patient requests access to their PHI, or an accounting of disclosures of their PHI.

A CE is required to disclose PHI to HHS for the purposes of a compliance investigation, review, or enforcement action.

Tarasoff, Aurora, Newtown: Protecting the patient and public from harm

In the wake of the mass shootings that occurred in Aurora, CO and Newtown, CT in 2012, the OCR issued a letter in January 2013 that provided guidance for healthcare providers regarding the ability to disclose information about a patient to law enforcement or others to protect the patient or the public from harm.

The duty to warn has its roots in the 1974 CA Supreme Court decision *Tarasoff v. the Regents of the University of California*,[3] which established a duty of healthcare providers to share warnings about credible threats of violence.

That duty was reaffirmed in the 2013 OCR letter,[4] which sought to balance patient privacy concerns with public health and safety:

When a healthcare provider believes in good faith that such a warning is necessary to prevent or lessen a serious and imminent threat to the health or safety of the patient or others, the Privacy Rule allows the provider, consistent with applicable law and standards of ethical conduct, to alert those persons whom the provider believes are reasonably able to prevent or lessen the threat.

---

[3] *Tarasoff v. Regents of the University of California*, 551 P.2d 334 (Cal. 1976).
[4] https://www.hhs.gov/sites/default/files/ocr/office/lettertonationhcp.pdf

Under these provisions, a healthcare provider may disclose patient information, including information from mental health records, if necessary, to law enforcement, family members of the patient, or any other persons who may reasonably be able to prevent or lessen the risk of harm.

The letter noted that most states have laws and/or court decisions supporting—even requiring—the disclosure of protected information in the interest of public safety, and recommends that healthcare providers consult state law as well as federal law governing the disclosure of substance abuse treatment records.

2.6 Minimum Necessary Standard

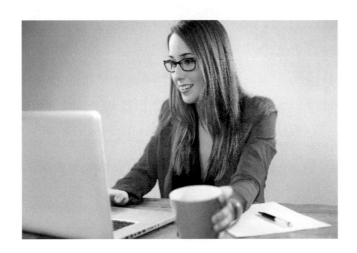

According to the HIPAA Privacy Rule, CEs cannot simply make any and all information available when using or disclosing PHI. The Privacy Rule exists to ensure that any PHI accessed by staff, shared, disclosed, or requested from another CE or BA is done in a mindful manner that protects the patient and safeguards confidentiality. This concept, known as the "minimum necessary standard," is a key protection of the Privacy Rule.

According to the standard, CEs are required to limit the use or disclosure of PHI to the minimum amount necessary to accomplish the intended purpose.

In the CE workplace, the standard means that workforce members who do not need to see patient PHI to do their jobs should not have access to it. It means that when a CE shares PHI with another CE or a BA, it only shares the information needed for that particular purpose.

For example, an entire patient history should not be shared to expedite payment for a specific treatment.

When implementing the minimum necessary standard, CEs are required to evaluate their practices to limit unnecessary or inappropriate access to PHI by determining which workforce members need access to PHI and under what conditions, based on job responsibilities and the nature of the business.

There are exceptions to the minimum necessary standard. It does not apply in the following situations:

- Disclosures to or requests by a healthcare provider for treatment purposes.
- Disclosures to the individual who is the subject of the information.
- Uses or disclosures authorized by the individual.
- Uses or disclosures required for HIPAA compliance.
- Disclosures to HHS when required for enforcement purposes.
- Uses or disclosures required by other laws, such as state laws.

2.7   Notice of privacy practices

A notice of privacy practices (NPP) is a statement that describes how the CE may use and disclose a patient's medical information, and the practices that the CE has implemented to keep PHI private. It also explains how patients can access their information and exercise their rights under HIPAA.

CEs are required by the Privacy Rule to draft an NPP in "plain language" and make it available to patients. The NPP must include the following information:

1. **A header.** The NPP must contain a header or a prominently displayed box containing this statement: "This Notice describes how medical information about you may be used and disclosed, and how you can get access to this information. Please review it carefully."

2. **How the CE may use and disclose PHI.** This section lists, with examples, all of the ways that the CE is permitted by HIPAA to use and disclose the patient's PHI.

3. **Uses and disclosures for additional activities.** If the CE uses PHI for fundraising, if it releases PHI to group health plan sponsors, or it uses PHI for underwriting purposes, it must include a statement describing those activities in a separate statement. With regard to underwriting, it must include language that says the CE is prohibited from using an individual's genetic PHI for this purpose. With regard to fundraising, it must inform the individual of the right to opt out of receiving such communications.

4. **The individual's rights with regard to PHI:**
   a. The right to request disclosure restrictions. The NPP should also include a statement that says the CE is not required to agree to requested restrictions, unless the patient pays for the services in full.
   b. The right to receive PHI through confidential communication.
   c. The right to request access.
   d. The right to request an amendment to the medical record.

    e.   The right to request an accounting of disclosures.

    f.   The right to request a paper copy of the NPP.

5.   **The CE's legal duties** with respect to the information, including statements that:

    a.   The CE is required by law to maintain the privacy of PHI.

    b.   The CE must notify patient impacted by a breach of unsecured PHI.

    c.   The CE reserves the right to change the terms of its NPP and explain how notice of the change will be provided to patients.

6.   **The individual's right to file a HIPAA complaint with the CE or the Secretary of HHS**, with instructions for filing the complaint, and a statement of non-retaliation.

7.   **Contact information** for individual (name or title and telephone number) who can provide further information about the CE's privacy policies.

8.   **The effective date of the NPP**, which cannot be retroactive.

A CE that has a direct treatment relationship with a patient must provide a copy of the NPP on the patient's first visit and make a good-faith effort to obtain a written acknowledgment of receipt from the patient.

NPP Templates

HHS has developed sets of model NPPs that health plans and healthcare providers can tailor and use for their operations. Each set contains three formatted options and a text-only option, in both English and Spanish:

https://www.hhs.gov/hipaa/for-professionals/privacy/guidance/model-notices-privacy-practices/index.html

In addition, the CE should make its NPP available to anyone who asks for it and post it prominently at its facility.

CEs that maintain a website with information about customer services or benefits must also post the NPP on the website.

The CE must promptly revise its NPP whenever it makes a change to its privacy practices, and must make patients aware of the changes by having copies available for patients to request and take with them, posting it in a prominent location at the facility, and on its website if it has one.

Are hospitals or other healthcare providers required to provide an NPP to patients they treat in an emergency?

No. A CE with a direct treatment relationship with an individual is not required to provide an NPP to a patient at the time of emergency treatment. In these situations, the HIPAA Privacy Rule requires only that providers give patients an NPP when it is practical to do so, after the emergency situation has ended.

The Privacy Rule also does not require that providers make a good-faith effort to obtain the patient's written acknowledgment of receipt of the notice if providing the NPP is delayed by an emergency treatment situation.

2.7.1.2 NPP acknowledgment of receipt

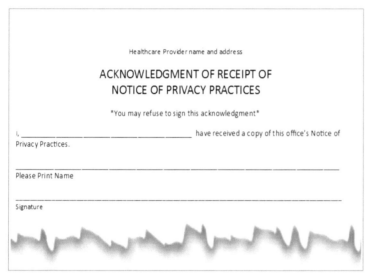

An acknowledgment of receipt is the form that patients are asked to sign on the first visit to acknowledge that they have received a copy of the NPP.

A CE with a direct treatment relationship with individuals is required to make a good-faith effort to obtain an individual's acknowledgement of receipt when the provider first gives the notice to the individual — that is, the first time that service is provided. An acknowledgment of receipt does not need to be signed by the patient each time.

What should a CE do if a patient refuses to sign an acknowledgment of receipt? The CE must try to get the patient to sign the receipt (and take the time to explain to the patient how the NPP works), but if an individual refuses to sign, the CE cannot compel them to sign, and cannot refuse to treat the patient simply because they have not signed the acknowledgment of receipt.

In addition, a patient's refusal to sign does **not** free the provider from complying with its privacy obligations. Staff should document efforts to obtain the patient's signature on the acknowledgment, and the reason why the acknowledgment was not signed.

2.8   The Rights of the Individual Under the HIPAA Privacy Rule

2.8.1 The right to access PHI

HIPAA provides individuals with the general right to access, inspect, and obtain a copy of their PHI for as long as the information is maintained by a CE or BA, regardless of the date it was created, the format of the PHI, or where the PHI originated. Individuals have the option of requesting a summary or explanation of the PHI. In addition, the right to access also allows individuals to direct a CE to share a copy of their PHI with a designated person or entity.

A CE must comply with a PHI request within 30 days. If that is not possible, the entity can obtain a 30-day extension by providing written notice (within the initial 30-day period) to the individual, with the reasons for the delay and the date that access will be provided.

2.8.2 The right to request restriction of uses and disclosures

Patients can ask CEs to restrict the use or disclosures of their PHI:

- For treatment, payment, or healthcare operations;
- To persons involved in the individual's healthcare or payment for healthcare; or
- To notify family members or others about the individual's general condition, location, or death.

For example, a patient may ask a care provider not to discuss treatment options if the patient's family is in the room.

2.8.3 The right to request confidential communications

A patient may have concerns about receiving telephone calls, texts, or mail from a CE regarding treatment or payment. HIPAA gives patients the opportunity to express those concerns to the CE. Patients have the right to specify how they would like the CE to communicate with them regarding their medical care and records.

For example, a patient may request that no messages be left on an answering machine, or that all correspondence be sent to a different address than the one listed on the patient's records.

2.8.4 The Right to request amendments of record

If a patient believes that PHI contained in a designated record set is incorrect, the patient can request that the PHI be amended. The CE has 60 days to respond to the request; it can take an additional 30 days if it notifies the patient in writing that it needs more time.

If the CE agrees to amend the PHI, it must capture the change in the patient's record and must make every effort to communicate the change to all individuals and entities that rely on that information for treatment purposes. The CE must also let the patient know that the requested amendment has been made.

When a CE amends a medical record and informs another CE or BA of the change, the CE receiving the information must also amend the patient's medical record.

2.8.5 The right to request an accounting of disclosures

A patient has the right to request information about disclosures of their PHI made by a CE or BA, with certain exceptions. This is called an accounting of disclosure. Patients can make these requests in writing or orally. If the request is made orally, the CE should document it on a general authorization form or a request for an accounting of disclosures form.

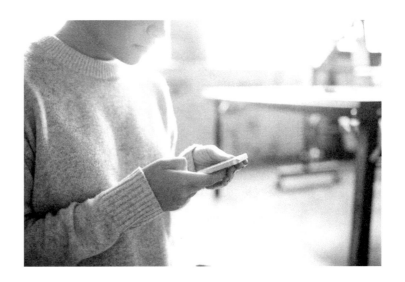

The CE must keep requests for accounting of disclosures with the patient's records, along with a copy of the written accounting provided to the patient. The accounting should also include the name of the person who provided the accounting.

When a patient makes a request for an accounting of disclosure, the request covers a maximum period of six years immediately preceding the accounting request (or a shorter time period if requested by the patient.)

When preparing the accounting of disclosures, the CE does not have to include disclosures made:

- For purposes of treatment, payment, or healthcare operations
- To the patient or personal representative
- To include the patient in a directory
- Pursuant to an authorization
- For national security purposes

- To correctional institutions/law enforcement agencies if related to an inmate or someone in custody

- As part of a limited data set

- Incidental disclosures permitted by the Privacy Rule

The CE must complete the accounting of disclosure within 60 days of the request. If the CE needs more time, it can get a 30-day extension if it provides the individual with a written statement explaining the delay and with the date that the accounting will be provided. The extension request must be made within the first 60 days.

2.8.6 The right to file a complaint

Patients have the right to complain if they believe that a CE or BA has committed a HIPAA Privacy Rule violation, or if they believe the CE or BA has not complied with its own privacy policies and procedures.

The CE must develop and implement a procedure that patients can use to file a complaint. The complaint procedure should include the following:

- A designated staff member who receives and processes complaints.

- Instructions for filing a complaint in the NPP. The instructions should include the name and position of the staff member designated to receive and process complaints, and should inform patients that they have the right to submit complaints directly to HHS. The instructions should also note that the CE cannot retaliate against the patient in any way for filing a complaint.

- A method to receive and document all complaints, such as using a complaint form to capture relevant information from the patient.

- Training staff on the proper way to handle a patient HIPAA complaint.

2.9   Privacy Rule Administrative Requirements

The HIPAA Privacy Rule requires CEs to develop a comprehensive plan to safeguard PHI and avoid prohibited uses and disclosures of the information. Entities that do not develop and implement a plan risk significant fines, costly corrective measures, and damage to their reputations.

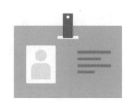

The Privacy Rule outlines the following administrative requirements:

1. Designate a privacy official

2. Train the workforce on privacy policies and procedures

3. Develop Privacy Rule safeguards

4. Develop a process for filing complaints

5. Establish sanctions for privacy violations

6. Make a mitigation plan

7. No retaliatory acts and no waiver of rights

8. Create policies and procedures for PHI protection

9. Develop a document management policy

2.10   The HIPAA Security Rule

The Security Rule complements the Privacy Rule, dealing specifically with ePHI.
It establishes a national set of security standards that CEs are required to implement in order to protect ePHI. The standards set forth safeguards to protect ePHI from internal and external threats, such as natural disasters, theft, unauthorized access, hacking, or phishing.

What are some key threats to data security?

- **Loss or damage of data due to a system crash, faulty equipment, or power failure**
- **Loss, corruption or theft of data by computer malware, hackers, or unauthorized users**
- **Loss or destruction of data due to a natural disaster, act of terrorism, or war**
- **User error**
- **Deliberate theft or damage by unscrupulous insiders**

At the same time, the Security Rule standards promote the appropriate access, sharing, and use of ePHI by healthcare entities to facilitate interoperability in healthcare operations. In fact, this is one of HIPAA's principal objectives, to support the adoption of industry-wide standards to manage ePHI. Legislators even included financial incentives in the Rule to drive faster adoption of the standards.

The Security Rule applies to health plans, healthcare clearinghouses, any healthcare provider that transmits health information in electronic form, and to BAs.

2.10.1 ePHI

Under the HIPAA Privacy Rule, PHI refers to all individually identifiable health information (IIHI) held or transmitted by a CE or BA in any form or media, including electronic, paper and oral.

The Security Rule protects that subset of PHI that a CE or BA creates, receives, maintains or transmits in electronic form. It does not apply to oral or paper PHI.

2.10.2 Overview of Security Rule Safeguards

The Security Rule applies to CEs such as health plans, healthcare clearinghouses, healthcare providers that transmit health information in electronic form, and BAs.

The Security Rule requires CEs and BAs to develop and implement safeguards to ensure the confidentiality, integrity, and availability of all ePHI created, received, maintained or transmitted.

Recognizing that information technology is constantly evolving, and that differently-sized entities require solutions tailored to their operations, the Rule does not specify the technologies that CEs must use. It is designed to be flexible, scalable and technology-neutral, allowing entities to identify the security measures that are the best fit for implementing the standards to protect ePHI. In determining which security measures and technologies are reasonable and appropriate for implementation, the entity should consider the following factors:

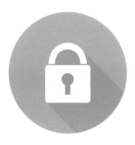

- Its size, complexity, and capabilities

- Its technical, hardware, and software infrastructure

- The costs of security measures

- The likelihood and possible impact of potential risks to ePHI

The Security Rule requires entities to implement administrative, physical, and technical safeguards. Each safeguard is made up of multiple standards that address specific situations within the safeguard. Most standards include implementation specifications, some required, some addressable, that provide more detailed guidance on how to implement the safeguard standard.

If an implementation specification is "required," the specification must be implemented. "Addressable" implementation specifications are not optional, but they give entities the flexibility to determine how to best implement safeguards tailored to their operations.

In meeting addressable specifications, entities must do one of the following:

- Implement the addressable specification;

- Implement one or more alternative measures that accomplish the same purpose; or

- Neither implement the addressable specification nor an alternative.

When making this decision, the entity should review factors such as its risk analysis, risk mitigation strategy, security measures currently in place, and the cost of implementation.

If an entity declines to implement an addressable specification, it must carefully document its decision and include the factors considered, including the results of the risk assessment.

2.10.3 Administrative Safeguards

Administrative safeguards are the administrative actions, policies, and procedures a CE or BA uses to select, develop, implement, and maintain security measures to protect ePHI. Administrative safeguards also include managing the entity's workforce with regard to protecting ePHI and monitoring the ongoing protection of the ePHI.

There are nine administrative safeguard standards established by the Security Rule, detailed below.

1. Security Management Process § 164.308(a)(1)	
This standard requires CEs and BAs to put policies and procedures in place to prevent, detect, contain, and correct security breaches. Potential threats to or possible vulnerabilities of ePHI must be identified and analyzed. Entities must continually evaluate the security system to ensure that it is operating according to established policies. Entities should conduct periodic security assessments to determine whether reasonable procedures are in place to protect against threats to the security or integrity of ePHI, as well as procedures to protect against reasonably anticipated uses or disclosures of ePHI by unauthorized personnel.	
Risk analysis (Required)	Entities are required to identify potential security risks to and vulnerabilities of all ePHI in their possession. To do this, entities must define how ePHI flows through the organization, track down less obvious sources of ePHI, such as portable devices, identify external sources of ePHI, and assess the human, natural, and environmental threats to information systems that contain ePHI.
Risk management (Required)	Entities must implement security measures to reduce risks and vulnerabilities. Entities can start by assessing the security measures already in place that are used to protect PHI, and then engage executive leadership in risk management and mitigation decisions, to ensure that security processes are being effectively communicated throughout the organization. Other resources that can be deployed to manage risk should also be identified.

Sanction policy (Required)	Entities must devise and apply sanctions against employees who do not comply with security policies and procedures. If an entity already has sanctions in place, those sanctions should be reviewed to ensure that they are sufficient to comply with this specification, or be modified as needed.

The sanctions policy should include examples of potential violations, and disciplinary action should match the severity of the violation. Employees should sign a statement that they agree to follow the entity's security policies and procedures, and that they understand that they are subject to disciplinary action if they violate them. |
| **Information system activity review (Required)** | Entities must develop and implement procedures to review information system activity, including audit logs, access reports, and security incident tracking reports. This review allows entities to determine whether ePHI has been used inappropriately.

Entities should examine existing information systems to determine whether the audit and review functions are robust, adequately used, and monitored. Logs and reports should be reviewed to ensure that they provide sufficient data on security. The entity must develop a policy to capture in detail how reviews will be conducted. |

2. Assigned Security Responsibility

This standard requires entities to designate a security official to be responsible for the development and implementation of the entity's policies and procedures.

The security official needs to have good working knowledge of the entity's IT operations in order to be able to create and implement an effective compliance plan to keep ePHI secure. The official is responsible for managing information security policies, procedures, and technical systems.

The designated officer's duties should be clearly identified, documented, and communicated to the officer, and those duties should properly reflect the entity's size and operations.

This standard does not have separate implementation specifications.

3. Workforce Security

This standard requires entities to implement policies and procedures that provide workforce members with job-appropriate access to ePHI, and to prevent unauthorized access to ePHI by workforce members who don't need access to ePHI to do their jobs.

The entity should identify workforce members who need access to ePHI to do their jobs, and specify the minimum necessary access needed for each job, as well as the computer systems and programs used to access ePHI. The next step is to implement policies and procedures that ensure only the identified individuals have access to the ePHI on specified computers, systems, and networks.

Authorization and/or supervision (Addressable)	Where reasonable and appropriate, entities must implement procedures to authorize and/or supervise individuals who work with ePHI, as well as computer systems that access ePHI. To perform this task, entities must designate someone to assign access permissions to ePHI and to develop job descriptions describing the access that different jobs have to ePHI. Entities may already have such rules in place for access to paper-based PHI, and can use those as a starting point for developing ePHI authorization and supervision processes.
Workforce clearance procedure (Addressable)	Where reasonable and appropriate, entities must implement procedures to ensure that workforce access to ePHI is authorized. Entities must provide and restrict access to ePHI in a meaningful way in order to ensure that designated workforce members have access to the information they need to do their jobs. Again, entities should start by examining processes already in place for paper PHI, and should check that procedures for determining access to ePHI are used consistently throughout the organization.
Termination procedures (Addressable)	Termination procedures (Addressable). Where reasonable and appropriate, entities must implement procedures for terminating access to ePHI when the relationship with an employee, contractor, or other individual ends, or when the individual or entity no longer requires access to ePHI. Termination policies must describe how an individual's access to ePHI will be restricted and the person responsible for terminating access. On the human resources side, there must be procedures in place to inform the person responsible for restricting ePHI access about such terminations in a timely manner.

Former employee costs CE more than $100,000 in HIPAA settlement[5]

A critical access hospital in Colorado agreed to pay a $111,400 settlement with OCR resulting from a complaint that a former Pagosa Springs Medical Center (PSMC) employee had continued to have remote access to the hospital's web-based scheduling calendar after ending their employment.

OCR determined that ePHI of 557 patients was disclosed without authorization to the former Pagosa Springs Medical Center (PSMC) employee.

The CE's failure to deactivate the former employee's access to all systems was a costly lesson in HIPAA compliance.

---

[5] https://www.hhs.gov/about/news/2018/12/11/colorado-hospital-failed-to-terminate-former-employees-access-to-electronic-protected-health-information.html

4. Information Access Management

This standard requires separating healthcare and clearinghouse services, and limiting access to ePHI to only those workforce members, contractors, and entities that need access. Procedures are needed for granting access that is consistent with a workforce member's need to work with ePHI. Access rights to specific workstations, transactions, programs, or processes should be clearly stated, documented, reviewed, and modified as necessary. In addition, when an individual leaves the organization or changes roles, their access to ePHI should be terminated or modified as appropriate.

As with the Workforce Security Standard, entities must take the Privacy Rule's minimum necessary requirements into account when developing and implementing policies and procedures to comply with this standard, in order to limit unnecessary or inappropriate access to and disclosure of protected health information. (See Section 2.6 on Minimum Necessary requirements.)

Entities are required to develop policies and procedures regarding the use of workstations, transactions, and software used to access ePHI. Entities should review permissions and modify them as needed.

Isolating healthcare clearinghouse functions (Required)	Healthcare clearinghouses that are part of a larger organization must implement policies and procedures that separate and protect the clearinghouse's ePHI from unauthorized access by the larger organization. In these cases, the clearinghouse must first determine whether the larger organization also performs healthcare clearinghouse functions, and if so, take care to also protect that ePHI from the larger organization's other operations. The clearinghouse should also check whether additional technical safeguards are needed to separate out ePHI in the clearinghouse's information systems, in order to prevent unauthorized access by workforce members from the larger organization.
Access authorization (Addressable)	Where reasonable and appropriate, entities must implement policies and procedures to grant ePHI access through devices and programs such as workstations, transactions, system programs, and processes. This safeguard complements the workforce security safeguard. Once an entity has determined who should have access to ePHI, it must determine how those individuals can access the information. The entity must develop policies and procedures that address how authorization is documented, and how it can be used to provide individuals with access to ePHI. Those policies and procedures must comply with Privacy Rule requirements. Access rules should be job-specific, and technical processes and conventions should be used to ensure appropriate access, such as creating unique user names and implementing an authentication process.
Access establishment and	Where reasonable and appropriate, entities are required to implement policies and procedures that establish, document, review, and modify user access to workstations, transactions, programs, and processes based on the policies and

modification (Addressable)	procedures developed for access authorization. Policies and procedures should be in place to set up and modify access privileges to ePHI, and those policies and procedures should be documented and updated as needed. The entity's security officer or another manager should periodically review who has access to ePHI and how access is controlled to ensure that policies and procedures are being properly implemented.

5. Security Awareness and Training

This standard requires entities to implement an ePHI security awareness and training program for all members of its workforce, including management.

Security safeguards only work if the people charged with implementing and following them understand why they exist, what the potential risks are, and what is expected of them.

Entities must provide comprehensive security training for all new and existing members of its workforce to make sure the workforce is ready and equipped to manage security issues. Workforce members should be retrained whenever external or internal changes happen that could affect ePHI security, such as updates to policies and procedures, updates to system hardware and software, or changes to the Security Rule or state laws.

Security reminders (Addressable)	Where reasonable and appropriate, entities must periodically update employees regarding changes to security policies and procedures. The entity can use the communication channels that are most effective for their workforce, such as printed or electronic notices, reminders on meeting agendas, and reminders posted around the workplace. Entities should also provide workforce members with periodic formal security retraining. All reminder and retraining activities must be documented.
Protection from malicious software (Addressable)	Where reasonable and appropriate, entities must implement procedures for protecting information systems from malicious software and for detecting and reporting malicious software incidents. Malicious software refers to viruses, Trojan horses, or worms designed to harm information systems. Bad actors can introduce malicious software (malware) in any number of ways, such as through email attachments or internet downloads, and use it to damage or destroy systems or to steal ePHI. Entities must continually educate workforce members about new threats and about their role in combatting malware attacks.
Login monitoring (Addressable)	Where reasonable and appropriate, entities must implement procedures to monitor attempts to log in to their information systems, and to report any suspected unauthorized login attempts.

	Most systems now incorporate login tracking as a basic capability. Smaller entities or entities with older systems should review their system capabilities to ensure that this specification is properly addressed.
Password management (Addressable)	Where reasonable and appropriate, entities must implement procedures to create, change, and protect passwords. Individuals should be trained on proper password practices, such as using strong passwords, safeguarding passwords, and never sharing passwords with others.

6. Security Incident Procedures

This standard requires entities to implement policies and procedures to address security incidents in a timely and effective manner. The Security Rule broadly defines a security incident as unauthorized access, use, disclosure, modification, or destruction of information or interference with system operations in an information system. Incidents include both attempted and successful breaches.

Entities should address all security incidents head on. Waiting to address an issue or attempting to conceal it will only exacerbate an already difficult situation. Detailed procedures should be developed and implemented to address suspected or known security incidents promptly. By taking immediate action, an entity may better mitigate the damage that occurs from a security incident.

The Security Rule requires entities to have a comprehensive plan to manage such incidents, starting with promptly determining whether an incident has occurred and a procedure for notifying the right people. The plan uses the results of the entity's risk analysis to be able to identify and respond to security incidents.

Response and reporting (Required)	Response and reporting (Required). Entities must immediately identify and respond to security incidents and take steps to mitigate harm that could result from the incident. Under the Privacy Rule, a BAA must include language that requires the BA to report security incidents to the CE.
	This specification requires entities to document all security incidents, measures taken to address them, and final outcomes. Entities should clearly communicate to workforce members the types of security incidents they may encounter, such as stolen passwords used to access ePHI; corrupted back-ups that result in the loss of ePHI; malicious software attacks; unauthorized access resulting from the use of a terminated employee's credentials; loss or theft of ePHI kept on laptops or mobile devices. Individuals must be trained on how to manage incidents, including reporting protocols, preserving evidence, and assisting with mitigation and documentation.

7. Contingency Plan

This standard requires entities to develop policies and procedures for responding to incidents that can hamper access to ePHI or damage information systems containing ePHI, such as power outages, fire, vandalism, system failure, and natural disasters. An entity's contingency plan must ensure that ePHI is protected at all times and available to authorized users.

Data backup plan (Required)	Entities must establish and implement procedures to create and maintain exact copies of ePHI that can be retrieved in the event of an emergency. Entities must identify all ePHI to be backed up, and determine the best back-up method, such as tape, disk, CDs, DVDs, or a secure cloud service, and ensure that backed-up ePHI is stored in a safe and secure location. The backup plan must include a back-up schedule designed to minimize information loss in the event of an emergency.
Disaster recovery plan (Required)	Entities must establish procedures to restore data lost during an emergency or other event. The recovery plan must be specific to the entity's operations and allow workforce members to identify the ePHI to be restored. The plan should be kept at multiple locations so that it can be implemented if the entity's location has been affected by an emergency.
Emergency mode operation plan (Required)	Entities must establish procedures that allow them to continue critical business processes that protect ePHI during an emergency. The plan should balance the need to access ePHI with the need to protect it during an emergency, and should include alternative security measures, including manual measures, to protect the ePHI. A contact list of all workforce members who should be notified in the event of an emergency, including their roles and responsibilities, should be kept with the plan.
Testing and revision procedures (Addressable)	Where reasonable and appropriate, entities must implement procedures to periodically test and revise contingency plans. The frequency and scope of the testing and revision procedures depend on a variety of factors, such as the complexity of the entity's organization, its size, and the costs of testing and revising plans. This specification applies to all plans made under the Contingency Plan Standard: the data backup plan, disaster recovery plan, and emergency mode operations plan. Entities should find ways to test plans, for example by using scenario-based walkthroughs, to ensure that the plans effectively address problems that could arise during an emergency. Testing should be used to ensure that all workforce members with responsibilities during an emergency understand their roles, and that they have participated in testing. Any problems discovered during testing should be addressed by revising plans as needed.
Applications and data criticality analysis (Addressable)	Where reasonable and appropriate, entities must evaluate the criticality of software applications used to store, maintain, and transmit ePHI for providing patient care and conducting business in order to prioritize emergency operations, back-up, and recovery. Entities should draft a prioritized list of specific applications and data to determine the order of restoration and to identify mission-critical applications.

8. Evaluation

This standard requires entities to perform technical and nontechnical evaluations to respond to environmental or operational changes that could affect the security of ePHI.

Entities can significantly increase their chances of successfully protecting ePHI by testing and evaluating the security safeguards they have put in place. The initial evaluation considers how the safeguards address Security Rule compliance; subsequent evaluations allow entities to examine real-world circumstances to help determine whether their security measures are adequate, and to identify needed changes.

The evaluation standard does not have separate implementation specifications.

9. Business Associate Contracts and Other Arrangements

This standard states that a CE may allow BAs to create, receive, maintain, or transmit ePHI on the its behalf only if the CE obtains satisfactory assurances from the BA that it will appropriately safeguard the information. Likewise, a BA may only use a third-party subcontractor to create, receive, maintain, or transmit ePHI on its behalf if it gets similar assurances from the subcontractor.

BAAs between the CE and its BAs must address HIPAA Privacy and Security Rules.

The BAA should require BAs to implement appropriate safeguards to prevent unauthorized use or disclosure of ePHI, and require BAs to report any use or disclosure of the information not provided for by its contract.

The CE should request and review BA security.

Written contract or other arrangement (Required)	CEs must document the assurances required by this standard with a written contract such as a BAA.

2.10.4 Physical Safeguards

Physical safeguards refer to the physical measures, policies, and procedures that an entity uses to protect electronic information systems, facilities, and equipment from natural and environmental hazards and from unauthorized access.

When implementing the physical safeguards, entities must take care to account for all of the ways that ePHI can be physically accessed, both inside the entity's facility and externally, for example, at the homes of employees or other places where they access ePHI.

The Security Rule has four physical safeguard standards.

1. Facility Access Controls

This standard requires entities to implement policies and procedures to limit physical access to information systems and to the interiors and exteriors of the facilities where the systems are kept, while at the same time allowing authorized personnel to access ePHI.

Contingency operations (Addressable)	Where reasonable and appropriate, entities must establish procedures that allow them to execute contingency plans created for the Contingency Plan Standard of the Administrative Safeguards. Physical access to facilities varies according to the entity's specific nature and operations. Entities should develop procedures that enable designated workforce members to be able to enter the facility to restore lost data or maintain access to ePHI in an emergency. The plan created for this specification should be included in the entity's contingency plan.
Facility security plan (Addressable)	Where reasonable and appropriate, entities must implement policies and procedures to keep the facility and equipment safe from unauthorized access, tampering, or theft. Physical access controls must ensure that only authorized persons can enter a facility, or specific areas of a facility that contain ePHI. Once the entity completes its risk assessment, the results can be used to develop a facility security plan that addresses any issues found in the assessment. Potential controls might include locked doors; use of key cards; surveillance cameras; alarms; restricted area signs; tags or engravings on computers and other property; visitor protocols; and a private security service.
Access control and validation procedures (Addressable)	Where reasonable and appropriate, entities must implement procedures to control and validate access to facilities based on employee roles or functions, including visitor control, and control of access to software programs for testing and revision. This specification should align with the facility security plan. It requires procedures to determine which workforce members have access to certain locations within the facility based on their role or function. Possible control measures include requiring proof of identity, key cards, and the use of visitor badges, as well as specific procedures to identify workforce members who are authorized to test and revise software. A list of individuals and their access rights should be included in the facility security plan.
Maintenance records (Addressable)	Where reasonable and appropriate, entities must implement policies and procedures to record repairs and modifications to the physical components of a facility that are related to security, such as changed hardware, repair or removal

of walls, doors, or locks, installing new security devices, and routine maintenance.

Entities can choose the type of maintenance record, such as log book, spreadsheet, or database, that works best for its size and operation. The record should include the following information: changes or repairs made; the date of the change; a description of the work done; who authorized the change; and who made the change or repair.

2. Workstation Use

This standard requires entities to identify the functions that are performed on computer workstations, such as what each workstation is used for, how it is used, and where it is located, in order to protect ePHI that is stored or used on the device.

This standard is designed to help entities avoid inappropriate use of computer workstations that could result in malicious software attacks and confidentiality breaches. Workstations are defined as any computing device, including laptops and desktop computers, electronic media and devices, tablets, mobile phones, servers, and network devices.

The policies and procedures developed for this standard must include policies that apply to workforce members with access to ePHI who work offsite or remotely. Common procedures include training all personnel to log off of their workstations when leaving their work areas, even for a short time, and cooperating with the IT department to make sure that antivirus software is up-to-date on all workstations.

The workstation use standard does not have separate implementation specifications.

3. Workstation Security

This standard requires entities to implement physical safeguards for all workstations with access to ePHI so that only authorized employees can use the workstations.

Entities must determine who is allowed access to workstations, and create physical safeguards to prevent unauthorized users from accessing or viewing ePHI on workstations. Measures include:

- Signs
- Physical barriers
- Designating a secure room as the only place where authorized personnel can access ePHI
- Positioning workstation screens away from areas from which they could be viewed
- Privacy screens to prevent others from viewing computer screens
- Cable locks to deter theft
- Port and device locks that physically restrict access to USB ports or CD/DVD drives (unrestricted access to USB ports and removable media devices can facilitate the unauthorized copying of data to removable media)

The physical safeguards used to protect workstations should be documented in the workstation use policies and procedures.

The workstation security standard does not have separate implementation specifications.

4. Device and Media Controls

This standard requires entities to implement policies and procedures to control and track the sale, transfer, or disposal of electronic media that is used to store, manage, or share ePHI. Electronic media includes memory devices in computers (hard drives) and any removable digital memory medium, such as magnetic tape or disk, optical disk, or digital memory card.

Disposal (Required)	Entities must implement policies and procedures to ensure the proper destruction and disposal of ePHI, including the process for making ePHI unusable and/or inaccessible, and of any hardware or electronic media that it is stored on.
Media re-use (Required)	Entities must implement policies and procedures that describe how ePHI is to be removed from electronic media before that media can be used again, to prevent unauthorized access.
Accountability (Addressable)	Where reasonable and appropriate, entities must track and document movement of ePHI from one location to another, including the person moving the ePHI. Laptop computers and mobile devices can be challenging to track. The individual responsible for tracking the movement of hardware and electronic media containing ePHI should perform an audit to identify all types of hardware and electronic media used, including laptops, mobile devices, thumb drives, optical disks, etc. The entity may want to assign tracking numbers to these devices and media to facilitate tracking efforts.
Data backup and storage (Addressable)	Where reasonable and appropriate, entities must create a retrievable, exact copy of ePHI, before moving hardware or electronic devices, if the entity considers that a copy is necessary. This specification protects the availability of ePHI and is similar to the data backup plan under the Administrative Safeguards that requires entities to create and maintain retrievable exact copies of ePHI. For example, an entity might decide to back up a hard drive before moving it, even though the data back-up plan does not include local hard drives. Entities could also provide employees with specific instructions about where ePHI files can be stored, such as designated folders on the network, eliminating the need for local hard drive back-ups.

2.10.5 Technical Safeguards

Technical safeguards are the technologies used to safeguard ePHI and the policies and procedures that address implementation of those technologies.

Entities use technical safeguards to prevent unauthorized access to ePHI inside and outside of the facility, to maintain the integrity of ePHI, and to track all access.

There are five technical safeguard standards established by the Security Rule.

1. Access Controls	
This standard requires CEs to implement technical policies and procedures to allow access to information systems containing ePHI to only those persons or software programs that have been granted access rights as specified in the Information Access Management standard. Access is the ability to read, write, modify, or communicate data, to or use a system resource. The access controls standard requires entities to set up a system of rights and permissions to control access to ePHI. The entity must apply the minimum necessary standard to only allow authorized users to access the ePHI necessary to perform their duties, and no more. (See Section 2.6 for Minimum Necessary Standard.)	
Unique user identification (Required)	Entities must assign each workforce member a unique name and/or number to be able to track all ePHI activity by user, and to identify responsible parties in the event of an ePHI security incident. Entities can set up their own naming convention, for example, a combination of first and last names. Many entities opt to use randomly assigned user identifiers made up of letters, numbers, and symbols because they are more difficult to hack (although they may also be more difficult for workforce members to remember). Trained IT personnel can help devise strategies that work best for the entity and comply with the requirements of the specification.
Emergency access procedure (Required)	Entities must establish ways their technology can be used to access ePHI in an emergency. The entity must specify exact practices that designated workforce members can use to get into the system in an emergency.
Automatic logoff (Addressable)	Where reasonable and appropriate, entities must implement procedures that automatically log a workstation off after a specified time of inactivity. Workforce members should be trained to log off of their workstations when they are finished working. Automatic logoff provides an extra safeguard in case an individual forgets to log off.

Encryption and decryption (Addressable)	Where reasonable and appropriate, entities must encrypt and decrypt ePHI. Encryption is process of making content unreadable by converting regular text into coded text. Proper use of encryption can prevent unauthorized users from viewing ePHI in a usable form, and can substantially reduce the risk of compromising ePHI.
	Encrypted data involved in a security incident is not considered unsecured ePHI, so breach notification to individuals and HHS is not required (See Chapter 6). This makes a compelling argument for implementing encryption safeguards, even though it is not a required implementation specification.

2. Audit Controls

This standard requires entities to implement hardware, software, and/or procedural mechanisms to record and inspect activity in information systems that contain or use ePHI.

Audit controls allow entities to track authorized access and identify potentially unauthorized access to ePHI. These controls are especially valuable when determining whether a security violation occurred. While the standard does not identify data that must be recorded or how often activity should be reviewed, an entity must consider its risk analysis and organizational factors, such as current technical infrastructure, hardware, and software security capabilities, in determining reasonable and appropriate audit controls.

Audit controls can include user activity and access accountability; access and modification of ePHI; log access; and fault logs to detect system errors.

The audit controls standard does not have separate implementation specifications.

3. Integrity

This safeguard standard requires entities to implement policies and procedures to protect ePHI from being altered or destroyed without authorization. These changes can result in clinical quality problems and patient safety issues.

Incidental or intentional changes or destruction of ePHI can be made by workforce members or BAs, and unauthorized changes can also occur without human intervention, for example due to electronic media errors or failures.

Entities must use tools that can confirm that ePHI has not been modified, falsified, or destroyed without authorization.

Mechanism to authenticate ePHI (Addressable)	Where reasonable and appropriate, entities must implement system tools and applications that can verify ePHI has not been altered or destroyed without authorization. The tools and applications should be tailored to address potential risks to the entity's ePHI

4. Person or Entity Authentication

This standard requires CEs to implement tools and procedures to verify the identity and authorization of a person or entity who is trying to access ePHI.

Entities need to know and be able to verify that users or other systems are who they say they are, and have authorized access to ePHI. CEs can use unique identifiers to authenticate users, such as passwords, secret words, photo IDs, tokens, badges, or biometric identifiers.

The person or entity authentication standard does not have separate implementation specifications.

5. Transmission Security

This standard requires CEs to implement technical security measures to protect ePHI from unauthorized access transmitted over an electronic communications network. The entity must review the methods of transmission, such as whether ePHI is sent through email, over the internet, or through some form of private or point-to-point network. Appropriate measures to protect ePHI as it is transmitted must be identified, implemented and documented.

Integrity controls (Addressable)	Where reasonable and appropriate, entities must implement security measures to ensure that electronically transmitted ePHI cannot be improperly modified without detection until disposed of.
	The integrity standard discussed in the third technical safeguard requires entities to protect ePHI that is stored in information systems. This implementation specification focuses on keeping ePHI from being changed or corrupted during transmission. Entities typically rely on network communication protocols to ensure that the data sent is the same as the data received. The entity's security officer should work closely with its IT department and vendor to address integrity controls.
Encryption (Addressable)	Where reasonable and appropriate, entities should encrypt ePHI before it is transmitted. This implementation specification is different from the encryption specification described in the Access Control standard (see Section 5.5.1) because it applies to encryption of ePHI in transit.
	Although the use of encryption is an addressable implementation specification, depending on the entity's business practices, there may be significant risk that ePHI can be accessed by unauthorized entities while the ePHI is being transmitted. If the entity's risk analysis indicates that the entity's ePHI could be vulnerable during transmission, an entity must encrypt those transmissions.
	Entities should discuss encryption needs and methods with their IT team, vendors and BAs. They should periodically reevaluate any encryption measures used to address possible changes in technology and newly emerging threats.

2.10.6 Organizational, Policies and Documentation Requirements

In addition to administrative, physical, and technical safeguards, the Security Rule includes four standards that define the organizational, policies and procedures, and documentation requirements of the Rule.

1. Business Associate Contracts or Other Arrangements

This standard requires CEs to have contracts or other arrangements with BAs that have access to the CE's ePHI. The standard specifies what must be included in a BAA.

This standard has one implementation specification for BA contracts. The CE and BA must enter into a BAA specifying that the BA will ensure that any of its subcontractors that handle a CE's ePHI on its behalf will enter into a contract with the BA that also requires compliance with HIPAA. The BAA must also require the BA to report any security incidents, including breaches of unsecured PHI, that it becomes aware of to the CE. Lastly, a BA and its subcontractor must enter into a contract similar to the BAA.

2. Requirements for Group Health Plans

This standard requires CEs that are group health plans to require the plan sponsor to safeguard ePHI that it creates, receives, maintains, or transmits on behalf of the plan.

The requirements for the group health plans standard has one required implementation specification that sets out the requirements for the plan documents of the group health plan. These plan documents must include provisions that require the plan sponsor to:

1. Implement administrative, technical, and physical safeguards for ePHI that the sponsor creates, receives, maintains, or transmits on behalf of the group plan;

2. Implement appropriate security controls to ensure adequate separation between plan sponsor employees who use and disclose ePHI;

3. Ensure that other parties that receive ePHI from the plan sponsor agree to protect ePHI by implementing appropriate security measures; and

4. Report all security incidents it becomes aware of to the group health plan.

3. Policies and Procedures

The Security Rule requires entities to document and create written policies and procedures for nearly every administrative, physical, and technical safeguard requirement. While this standard requires entities to implement reasonable and appropriate policies and procedures, it does not define the exact content or format. The Rule's flexibility and scalability permit entities to determine how to address these tasks and tailor them to their own size and business type in order to reflect the entity's mission and culture. This standard is further supported by the Documentation standard.

4. Documentation	
This standard requires entities to document the policies and procedures that they implement to comply with the Security Rule. Any action, activity, or assessment taken by the entity in order to comply with the Security Rule must also be documented. The entity can keep paper or electronic records to document policies, procedures, and other related activities.	
Time Limit (Required)	Entities must retain the documentation of all policies and procedures for a minimum of six years from the date of their creation or the date when they were last in effect, whichever is later. Entities may opt to keep their documentation for longer periods of time based on state law or for other business reasons.
Availability (Required)	Entities must make documentation available to those persons responsible for implementing procedures, such as making documentation available in printed or electronic manuals.
Updates (Required)	Entities must periodically review documentation and make appropriate updates in response to environmental or operational changes affecting the security of ePHI.

2.11 Reporting Non-Compliance

What should an employee do if they suspect non-compliance with the Security Rule? They should report it **immediately** to the designated security official, with full confidence that there will be no retaliation for making the report.

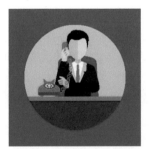

If the security official finds that there is a possible breach, i.e. an impermissible use or disclosure of ePHI, he or she would launch the breach notification protocol.

When dealing with a possible breach, the official should automatically assume there has been a breach, unless the circumstances meet one of these breach exceptions:

- There was unintentional access, use or acquisition of ePHI
- The disclosure was between two authorized people
- The disclosure was made by a CE or BA, and there is a good- faith belief that unauthorized person was not likely to retain the information
- A risk assessment finds that there is a low level of compromise

A risk assessment will consider these factors to determine the level of compromise:

- The nature and extent of ePHI involved, including the likelihood of re-identification

- The unauthorized person who used the ePHI or to whom the disclosure was made
- Whether the ePHI was actually acquired or viewed
- The extent to which the risk to the ePHI has been mitigated

2.12   Breach Notification Rule

A CE is required to notify affected individuals of any unauthorized access, use, disclosure or acquisition of unsecure ePHI without reasonable delay and within 60 days of the discovery via first class mail. (Some states require notification within 30 days—security officials should check their state statutes.)

Under this Rule, a breach is broadly defined as an impermissible use or disclosure of unsecured PHI that compromises the affected individuals' security or privacy. Unsecured PHI is PHI that has not been made unusable, unreadable, or indecipherable through encryption or destruction.

If a CE discovers a breach of unsecured PHI, and a risk assessment indicates that there is more than a low probability that the PHI is compromised, the Breach Notification Rule requires the CE to notify affected individuals.

CEs must also notify the HHS Secretary of any unsecured PHI breaches. If a breach affects 500 or more individuals, the CE must notify HHS as quickly as reasonably possible, and no later than 60 days after the discovery of a breach. If a breach affects fewer than 500 individuals, the CE can notify HHS in an annual report. A breach of this size must be reported no later than 60 days after the end of the calendar year in which it is discovered.

The CE must also alert the major media outlets in the region if the breach affects more than 500 people. It must post information about the breach and contact information on its website for 90 days if it is unable to contact more than 10 of the affected individuals.

HHS maintains an online breach portal, unofficially known as the "Wall of Shame," where it publishes a list of entities that have experienced breaches that have affected 500 or more people. Strict adherence to the Security Rule and continuous review of HIPAA policies and procedures are critical to ensuring entities stay off this website

2.12.1 Breach by a BA

If a BA discovers a breach of ePHI, it must notify the CE immediately. The CE is typically responsible for notifying affected individuals. However, notification can be the BA's responsibility if it is included in the BAA.

The 7 Steps to Address a HIPAA Complaint

Timely Respond to Patient Complaints

The clock is ticking if there is a breach of PHI. Penalties can be avoided/reduced if corrected within

30 DAYS

Conduct an Adequate Investigation

Correct and Mitigate Harmful Effects

Determine if there is a Reportable Breach

Do not report if an exception applies:

- Unintentional access that does not result in further use or disclosure that violates HIPAA.
- An inadvertent disclosure of PHI
- Good faith belief that the unauthorized person would not likely retain the PHI

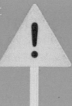

Report the breach If there is more than a low probability of PHI compromise based on a risk assessment of the 4 factors:

- The nature and extent of the PHI involved, including the types of identifiers and the likelihood of re-identification
- The unauthorized person who used the PHI or to whom the disclosure was made
- Whether the PHI was actually acquired or viewed
- The extent to which the risk to the PHI has been mitigated

Involve HR to Determine Disciplinary Measures

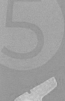

HIPAA requires covered entities to sanction employees who violate HIPAA. Work with HR to identify the appropriate disciplinary measures to take.

Follow up with the Patient

Notify the patient of the findings and resolution of their complaint.

Document and Record all Investigative Efforts

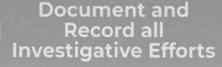

Click here for a sample HIPAA Privacy Complaint Form.

Comprehensive Healthcare Compliance Management Solutions

CONFIDENCE INCLUDED

Creating confidence among compliance professionals through education, resources, and support

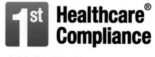
1st Healthcare® Compliance

888.54.FIRST 1sthcc.com

2.13   The HIPAA Enforcement Rule

The HIPAA Enforcement Rule contains provisions for HIPAA compliance and investigations, provisions for imposing monetary penalties for HIPAA Privacy and Security violations, and provisions for hearings procedures.

A number of federal agencies are involved in enforcing HIPAA regulations:

The Office for Civil Rights (OCR). The OCR is charged with protecting health information privacy rights. The agency investigates health information privacy and patient safety confidentiality complaints. It also engages in education activities for health and social service workers and community members about health information privacy and patient safety confidentiality laws.

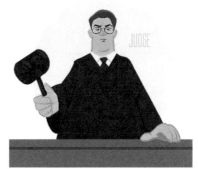

Center for Medicare and Medicaid Services (CMS). CMS works with healthcare providers, health plans and clearinghouses to help them with HIPAA compliance through education and complaint-driven enforcement. CMS has the authority to investigate HIPAA complaints and perform audit compliance for transactions, code sets, unique identifiers and operating rules.

Department of Justice (DOJ). The OCR works in conjunction with the (DOJ) to investigate and impose consequences for criminal violations of HIPAA.

Pursuant to the HITECH Act, enforcement authority is also granted to States Attorney General to bring civil actions on behalf of state residents for violations of the HIPAA Privacy and Security Rules.

2.13.1 HIPAA enforcement and penalties

OCR HIPAA enforcement activity consists of conducting compliance reviews of CEs and BAs, as well as investigating HIPAA complaints filed with the agency.

When a compliance review, notification of a breach, or HIPAA complaint reveals that a CE is in noncompliance, OCR will typically first try to work with the entity to resolve the issue. Possible outcomes include voluntary compliance by the CE, corrective action, or a resolution agreement.

HIPAA violations can also result in civil and criminal penalties. If a review or complaint reveals activity that could be a violation of the criminal provisions of HIPAA (violations that were committed "knowingly"), OCR may refer the complaint to the DOJ for investigation.

2.13.1.1 Civil monetary penalties

For non-criminal violations, if the CE does not resolve the matter to the OCR's satisfaction, the agency may impose civil monetary penalties.

The Enforcement Rule uses a four-tiered civil penalty structure. The HHS Secretary has discretion in determining the amount of the penalty, based on the type and extent of the violation and the harm resulting from the violation. Penalties for willful neglect are mandatory.

The Secretary takes any corrective action taken by the CE into account, and cannot impose civil penalties (except in cases of willful neglect) if the violation is corrected within 30 days. HHS has the authority to extend this time period.

This penalty tier structure was released in a Notification of Enforcement by the Department of Health and Human Services (HHS) on April 30, 2019, and will be adjusted for inflation. The Federal Civil Penalties Inflation Adjustment Act Improvements Act of 2015 directs agencies such as the HHS to adjust civil monetary penalties (CMPs) for inflation based on a prescribed formula. New CMP amounts are published annually in the Federal Register.

HIPAA Violation	Minimum Penalty	Annual Limit
Unknowing	$100 per violation	$25,000
Reasonable Cause	$1,000 per violation	$100,000
Willful neglect but violation is corrected within the required 30-day time period	$10,000 per violation	$250,000
Willful neglect and is not corrected within required time period	$50,000 per violation	$1,500,000

2.13.1.2 Criminal penalties

Criminal violations of HIPAA are handled by the DOJ. Like the OCR, the DOJ imposes criminal penalties of varying severity depending upon the nature and the extent of the violation. Criminal penalties include monetary penalties and imprisonment.

HIPAA CEs that knowingly obtain or disclose PHI can face a fine of up to $50,000, as well as imprisonment up to 1 year. That fine will increase to $100,000 and five years in prison if the DOJ finds that the offense was committed under false pretenses.

If an offense is committed with the intent to sell, transfer, or use PHI for commercial advantage, personal gain, or malicious harm, a fine of up to $250,000 could be imposed, along with and up to 10 years of imprisonment.

HIPAA Violation	Monetary Penalty	Prison Sentence
Knowingly obtain or disclose PHI	$50,000	Up to 1 year in prison
Using, obtaining or disclosing PHI under false pretenses	$100,000	Up to 5 years in prison
Intent to use PHI for advantage, gain, or harm	$250,000	Up to 10 years in prison

What did you learn? Discussion topics for Chapter 2

➢ What is the difference between a covered and a non-covered entity?

➢ What are some examples of protected health information (PHI)?

➢ Why do healthcare providers need patients to sign an Acknowledgement? What happens if a patient does not want to sign?

➢ What are the three types of safeguards that healthcare providers must use to comply with the Security Rule? Describe each safeguard.

➢ What must a healthcare provider do if there is an unauthorized disclosure of PHI?

➢ What is the most serious category of HIPAA violations? What are the civil and criminal penalties for those violations?

Online Resources

"HIPAA Enforcement." This webpage summarizes HIPAA enforcement procedures, including links to case examples. https://www.hhs.gov/hipaa/for-professionals/compliance-enforcement/

5 Common HIPAA Compliance Myths

Myth #1

"I don't bill Medicare, so I don't need to follow HIPAA Rules"

All covered entities must abide by HIPAA Privacy and Security Rules. Covered entities include healthcare providers, health plans and healthcare clearing houses. Only healthcare providers who do not transmit claims electronically meet an exception.

Myth #2

"As the patient, I own my whole medical record and I want it now."

HIPAA allows individuals the Right to Access and to receive a copy of the Designated Record Set within 30 days. However, the patient does not have ownership of the entire medical record. The provider "owns" the medical record.

Myth #3

"While looking up a patient on the EHR, I accidentally looked up the wrong patient. This is a breach and it needs to be reported."

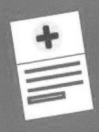

Not every impermissible use or disclosure is considered a breach. Under HIPAA, there are exceptions to what is a true breach requiring breach notification, such as in this case. Keep in mind that if the impermissible use or disclosure does not meet one of the exceptions, there are strict deadlines to meet under the Breach Notification Protocol to avoid violations and subsequent penalties for untimely reporting.

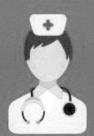

Myth #4

"Since it was my Business Associate, a billing company that caused the large breach of PHI, I am off the hook."

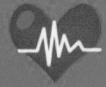

With a valid written Business Associate Agreement (BAA), this may be true in regard to the financial harm from penalties for a breach by the Business Associate, but this may not prevent significant reputational harm to the covered entity.

Myth #5

"In the waiting room, the nurse should not call out my name [PHI] when it's time to see the doctor."

This is an example of an Incidental Use which is permitted by HIPAA. However, there are many ways that PHI may be impermissibly disclosed from your facility. An unsuspecting employee can easily be the source of a breach of PHI by simply opening or sending an email.

Creating confidence among compliance professionals through education, resources, and support

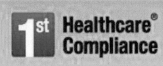

"HIPAA Security Series #4: Security Standards: Technical Safeguards." The fourth paper explores the standards for Technical Safeguards and their implementation specifications. https://www.hhs.gov/sites/default/files/ocr/privacy/hipaa/administrative/securityrule/techsafeguards.pdf

"HIPAA Security Series #5: Security Standards: Organizational, Policies and Procedures and Documentation Requirements." The fifth paper looks at the standards for Organizational Requirements and Policies and Procedures and Documentation Requirements. https://www.hhs.gov/sites/default/files/ocr/privacy/hipaa/administrative/securityrule/pprequirements.pdf

"HIPAA Security Series #6: Security Standards: Basics of Risk Analysis and Risk Management.**"** The sixth paper considers required risk analysis and risk management implementation specifications. https://www.hhs.gov/sites/default/files/ocr/privacy/hipaa/administrative/securityrule/riskassessment.pdf

"HIPAA Security Series #6: Security Standards: Implementation for the Small Provider.**"** The seventh paper considers implementation of the Security Rule standards, implementation specifications and requirements as they relate to CEs that are sole practitioners or otherwise considered small providers.https://www.hhs.gov/sites/default/files/ocr/privacy/hipaa/administrative/securityrule/small provider.pdf

Chapter 3

OSHA

Overview

The Occupational Safety and Health Administration (OSHA) sets and enforces standards designed to ensure safe and healthful working conditions. In this chapter, you will learn about the OSHA standards that healthcare employers must comply with, as well as the possible consequences of OSHA violations and a plan for compliance.

Chapter Outline

3.1   OSHA Background
3.2   OSHA Compliance Plan
3.3   OSHA Standards
3.4   OSHA Violations and Penalties

Learning Objectives

After completing this chapter, you should be able to do the following:

✓   Explain the significance of OSHA, the OSHA employer responsibilities, and employee rights.
✓   Name and understand the basic components of an OSHA compliance plan.
✓   List the nine OSHA standards that apply to the healthcare industry.
✓   Name the six classes of OSHA violations and the corresponding penalties.
✓   List the OSHA violations that occur most frequently in healthcare settings.

3.1 OSHA Background

The Occupational Safety and Health Administration (OSHA) is an agency of the US Department of Labor that was established by Congress under the Occupational Safety and Health Act and signed into law by President Richard Nixon in 1970. The passage of the Act and creation of the agency were a direct response to the growing number of workplace accidents at the time.

OSHA only addresses employee safety! Patient safety is not regulated under OSHA.

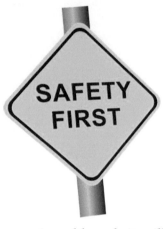

OSHA's mission is to "assure safe and healthful working conditions for working men and women by setting and enforcing standards and by providing training, outreach, education and assistance." The agency seeks to fulfill this mission of protecting workers by encouraging both employers and employees to reduce workplace hazards, and improve existing or implement new safety and health programs.

OSHA standards apply to most employers in all U.S. jurisdictions (the 50 states and the District of Columbia) through federal OSHA or OSHA-approved state plans. OSHA also applies to all federal agencies, although it will not impose fines on them; it will merely conduct inspections in response to complaints.

State and local government workers are not covered by OSHA. They are protected if they work in one of the 22 states with an OSHA-approved program.

Workers who are self-employed, and farmers and their family members are not covered by OSHA.

3.1.1 General duty clause: Employer responsibilities

All employers must comply with OSHA standards. Under the OSHA General Duty Clause, employers are required to provide a workplace free of recognized hazards that are causing or are likely to cause death or serious physical harm to employees. Employers must:

- Find and correct safety hazards and sources of health problems

- Make changes to improve working conditions

- Minimize risks by using safer chemicals for cleaning, trapping harmful fumes with enclosures, or using ventilation systems to clean the air

- Develop mandatory job safety standards and enforce them

- Provide research and development for better, safer ways to deal with occupational safety issues, including input from the employees

- Maintain a recording and record-keeping system and procedure to monitor job-related injuries and illness

- Establish training programs for personnel

3.1.2 Employee rights

Under OSHA, employees have the right to a safe workplace. This includes:

- A workplace free of known safety and health hazards

- Information about possible hazards or dangers present in the workplace

- Safe machinery

- Training on ways to prevent harm, in language that is easily understood

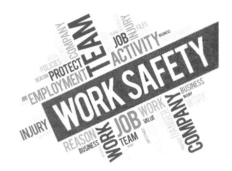

- Appropriate safety gear

- Protection from toxic chemicals

- Access to the workplace injury and illness log

- Access to the results of tests performed to find potential workplace hazards

- The ability to report a work-related injury or illness

- The ability to voice concerns and/or request an OSHA inspection without fear of retribution

An employee who believes he or she is working in an unsafe environment has the right to take the following actions:

- File a complaint with OSHA
- Request an OSHA inspection of the workplace
- Speak with an OSHA inspector privately during the investigation

An employee has the right to take these actions without having to fear retribution or retaliation by the employer.

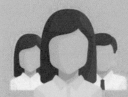
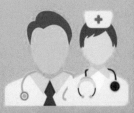

10 Common OSHA Violations in the Healthcare Setting

1 Failure to implement and maintain an exposure control program under BPP Standard

2 Failure to train under BPP Standard

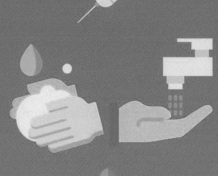

3 Failure to engineer out hazards / ensure hand washing under BBP Standard

4 Poor housekeeping under BBP Standard

5 Failure to implement and maintain a written Hazard Communication Program

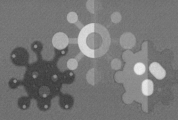

6 Failure to make the Hepatitis B vaccination available under BBP Standard

7 Failure to prepare exposure determinations under BBP Standard

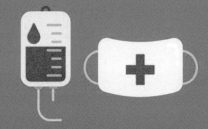

8 Failure to use personal protective equipment under BBP Standard

9 Failure to provide post exposure Hepatitis B vaccination under BBP Standard

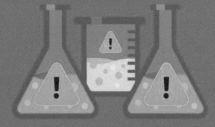

10 Failure to train employees under Hazard Communications Standard

To avoid potential areas of noncompliance regularly audit your practice for safety and health hazards. Employee training and periodic refresher training is essential, especially regarding Bloodborne Pathogen and Hazard Communication education.

Comprehensive Healthcare Compliance Management Solutions

CONFIDENCE INCLUDED

Creating confidence among compliance professionals through education, resources, and support

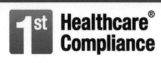 **1st Healthcare® Compliance**

888.54.FIRST 1sthcc.com

There is zero tolerance for discrimination and retaliation for filing an OSHA complaint. If an employee feels discriminated against after the employer receives notification of OSHA inspection prompted by the employee's complaint, or if the employee believes that his or her OSHA rights have been compromised or he or she is being punished for being a "whistleblower," the employee can file a complaint directly with OSHA.

3.2   OSHA Compliance Plan

Every healthcare office is required to develop and execute an OSHA compliance plan. This plan must be reviewed and updated at least once a year. Employees must receive training on the plan and on any changes made to the plan.

The OSHA compliance plan should clearly identify the safety coordinator or OSHA compliance officer for the organization. At the very least, the plan should include policies and procedures regarding the nine OSHA standards most applicable to the healthcare industry:

- Hazard Communication Standard
- Bloodborne Pathogens Standard
- Ionizing Radiation Standard
- Exit Route Standard
- Electrical Safety Standard
- Emergency Action Plan Standard
- Fire Safety Standard
- Medical First-Aid Standard
- Personal Protective Equipment Standard

Other OSHA standards and regulations that should be considered for a compliance plan include:

- General Housekeeping
- Ergonomics
- Workplace Violence Prevention

 An OSHA compliance plan should not be a generic off-the-shelf plan. It must be a plan that is tailored to the needs and operations of the individual organization or workplace.

3.3   OSHA Standards

Under the Occupational Safety and Health Act, OSHA has the authority to issue workplace health and safety regulations, known as OSHA Standards. These standards regulate the methods that employers must use to address the employee rights described in Section 3.1.

There are nine OSHA standards that are most frequently addressed with regard to the healthcare industry. Healthcare providers must take each of these standards into account when developing an OSHA compliance plan. This section discusses each standard in detail.

3.3.1 The hazard communication standard

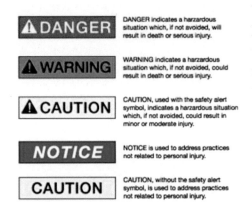

Under this OSHA standard, workers have a right to know and understand about any possible hazards in their workplace. This means that employers are required to provide employees with access to information about hazards in their workplace and how to protect themselves. Since the Hazard Communication Standard was instituted, the number of workplace injuries and illnesses due to chemical exposure has been cut almost in half.

The Hazard Communication Standard originally gave employees the "right to know" about workplace hazards, but it was revised in 2012 to give employees the "right to understand." This change came as OSHA aligned the standard to the United Nations' Globally Harmonized System of Classification and Labeling of Chemicals.

The revised standard, known as HAZCOM2012, addressed the following:

- Hazardous material classification
- Practices for labeling hazardous products
- Safety data sheet requirements
- Information and employee training requirements

The deadline for compliance with the U.N. system for all end users was June 1, 2016.

3.3.1.1 The OSHA 6-step hazard communication program

OSHA offers six steps for developing and implementing an effective hazard communication program:

3.3.1.1.1 Designate a staff member to lead the program

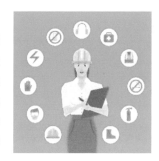

Select an individual to prepare and implement the hazard communication program, and notify employees. All employees must know who the program coordinator is. Although specific tasks (such as maintaining safety data sheets or ensuring that labels on containers received from vendors are compliant) may be assigned to other individuals, the program coordinator is ultimately responsible for ensuring compliance with the standard.

3.3.1.1.2 Prepare and implement a written hazard communication program

The program coordinator must develop a written hazard communication program that provides employees with information on workplace hazards before the employee begins any work that may involve those hazards, and when any new hazards are identified. The program should include a list of all hazardous chemicals that employees may be exposed to and guidance on how to protect themselves from chemical exposure. The list can be organized in the best manner suited for the size of the business.

3.3.1.1.3 Ensure containers of hazardous materials are correctly labeled

Hazardous chemical containers must have labels prepared and affixed by the manufacturers and suppliers. The labels must be in English, clearly displayed, and provide complete hazard information and precautionary measures. Warnings can be added in other languages if necessary. Additional information will be included on the companion Safety Data Sheet.

Hazardous chemical labels must include the following information:

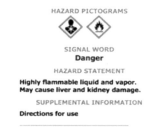

Product identifier

► Chemical name, code number or batch number used to identify the hazardous chemical
► Designated by the manufacturer, importer or distributor designate
► The identifier on the label must match the identifier found in section 1 of the corresponding Safety Data Sheet for that chemical

Signal word

► A word that indicates the relative level of hazard severity to alert the reader. For example: Danger—more severe; Warning—less severe
► Only the word indicating the highest danger level should appear

HAZARD PICTOGRAMS

SIGNAL WORD
Danger

HAZARD STATEMENT

**Highly flammable liquid and vapor.
May cause liver and kidney damage.**

SUPPLEMENTAL INFORMATION

Directions for use

_____

_____

Hazard statements

▶ These statements are specific classification categories that describe the nature of the hazard, for example "toxic if swallowed"

▶ The statements may also include the degree of the hazard.

▶ Statements on a single product may be combined to reduce redundancies and improve readability, but they must include specific hazard information

---

HAZARD PICTOGRAMS

SIGNAL WORD
Danger

HAZARD STATEMENT

**Highly flammable liquid and vapor.
May cause liver and kidney damage.**

SUPPLEMENTAL INFORMATION

Directions for use

_____

Pictograms

▶ There are 9 standard OSHA pictograms to alert users about chemical hazards. Labels must include the appropriate pictogram

▶ The red diamond on a white background frames a hazard symbol to specify the hazard type

▶ The Department of Transportation also uses diamond-shaped symbols on transport containers

---

SUPPLIER IDENTIFICATION

Company Name _____
Street Address _____
City _____ State _____
Postal Code _____ Country _____
Emergency Phone Number _____

PRECAUTIONARY STATEMENTS

Keep container tightly closed. Store in cool, well ventilated place that is locked.
Keep away from heat/sparks/open flame. No smoking.
Only use non-sparking tools.
Use explosion-proof electrical equipment.
Take precautionary measure against static discharge.
Ground and bond container and receiving equipment.
Do not breathe vapors.

Precautionary statements

▶ Precautionary statements list the measures users should take to minimize or prevent adverse effects from exposure to a hazardous chemical or from improper storage or handling

▶ Statement are categorized as:
  - Prevention (wear protective gloves, wash hands after handling
  - Response (in case of a fire use water spray)
  - Storage (store in a cool, well ventilated, locked place)
  - Disposal (dispose container in accordance with regulations)

▶ Precautionary statements on labels must match statements on Safety Data Sheets.

PRODUCT IDENTIFIER

CODE _____
Product Name _____

SUPPLIER IDENTIFICATION

Company Name _____
Street Address _____
City _____ State _____
Postal Code _____ Country _____
Emergency Phone Number _____

PRECAUTIONARY STATEMENTS

Keep container tightly closed. Store in cool, well ventilated place that is locked.
Keep away from heat/sparks/open flame. No smoking.

Manufacturer/supplier information

▶ Accurate supplier identification is critical so that that a supplier can be reached in the event of an emergency.

▶ The supplier should include an emergency phone number in this section.

▶ According to the Globally Harmonized System, manufacturers must update any new information on labels and Safety Data Sheets within six months and distribute them to end users.

3.3.1.1.4 Maintain safety data sheets

Employers must maintain a Safety Data Sheet (SDS) for each hazardous chemical in the workplace. The SDS must use the 16-section SDS format developed by the Globally Harmonized System and adopted by OSHA with the revision of HAZCOM 2012. The 16 sections are:

1. Identification
2. Hazard(s) identification
3. Composition/information on ingredients
4. First-aid measures
5. Firefighting measures
6. Accidental release measures
7. Handling and storage
8. Exposure control/personal protection
9. Physical and chemical properties
10. Stability and reactivity
11. Toxicological information
12. Ecological information
13. Disposal considerations
14. Transport information
15. Regulatory information
16. Other information

Sections 12-15 are regulated by other agencies and not enforced by OSHA. The information must still be on the SDS.

The manufacturer or supplier of the hazardous chemical is required to provide the employer with a compliant SDS. If there are any changes to the information, the manufacturer or supplier must provide the employer with a revised SDS within six months.

SDS sheets should not be kept for hazardous chemicals that are no longer used in the facility, or for non-hazardous chemicals. For example, common household cleaning supplies that are used the same way that they are used at home are not covered under the Hazard Communication Standard, and do not need hazardous chemical labels or SDS.

The employer must establish procedures for handling a hazardous chemical that is received without an SDS. Employers must make a good faith effort to obtain an accurate SDS from the manufacturer or distributor, but workers should not use that chemical until a SDS has been received. If a manufacturer or supplier does not provide a missing SDS after it has been requested, the employer should contact OSHA for further assistance.

Employers ensure that employees have easy access to the Safety Data Sheets. Although OSHA does not have specific requirements regarding the way that employers should make SDS available, the agency is emphatic that SDS must be readily available to employees at all times.

Employers should keep hard copies of the SDS in a binder, and keep the binder on-hand and easily accessible. Electronic SDS are acceptable, but there must be a contingency plan and backup copy in the event of a power outage.

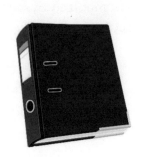

SDS must be in English. Other languages are also permitted if applicable.

3.3.1.1.5 Inform and train employees

Employers must develop a comprehensive training program and provide employees with annual training. Training content and materials must be up-to-date and aligned with the U.N. Globally Harmonized System of Classification and Labeling of Chemicals (GHS).

New employees must be informed about the hazardous chemicals they will potentially be exposed to during their workday, and receive additional training whenever there are changes to existing chemical hazards and/or new hazardous chemicals are brought into the workplace.

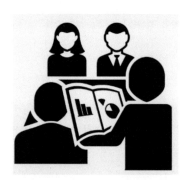

Employee training should include a detailed explanation of the GHS label requirements and the 16-section Safety Data Sheet format. Employees must also know where Safety Data Sheets are kept in the workplace so that they can get to them quickly in the event of an emergency or non-emergency. Training should also instruct on methods to detect the presence or release of hazardous chemicals, spell out any hazards, including physical, health, asphyxiation, combustible dust, pyrophoric gas, as well as appropriate protective measures.

Employers are not required to keep records of training activities, but the records could prove very useful in the event of an OSHA inspection.

3.3.1.1.6 Evaluate program

Employers should continuously evaluate the Hazard Communication Program to make sure it is working. The program should be revised to address any problems and updated whenever new information becomes available.

3.3.2 Bloodborne pathogen standard

Employers must protect workers who could be exposed to health hazards caused by bloodborne pathogens. Bloodborne Pathogens (BBPs) are organisms found in the blood or other potentially infectious materials. The most common BBPs are Hepatitis B, Hepatitis C, and HIV.

To protect workers, the BBP standard requires employers to develop and implement a written exposure control plan to prevent or reduce workplace exposure to BBPs. The plan should include an exposure determination list (EDL) containing job classifications that identify all jobs that expose employees to BBPs. The EDL should also include a detailed description of all employee tasks that could result in occupational exposure.

OSHA does not keep a list of safer devices.

The BBP standard was revised with the Needlestick Safety and Prevention Act in 2000, which requires employers to seek out and implement new, safer devices, such as sharps disposal containers and needleless systems in the workplace in order to minimize exposure risk.

Input from those employees at greatest risk of exposure should help drive device decisions. Annual plan revisions should include any updates to EDL and changes to policies and procedures. Employee input regarding the identification and adoption of safer techniques and new devices should be documented in the EDL.

3.3.2.1 Elements of an exposure control plan

- **Exposure determination list.** This is a detailed list of all job classifications, tasks and activities that could expose employees to BBPs.

  Employers do not need to provide a sharps container for syringes for a diabetic employee.

- **New techniques and devices, with employee input.** Employers must work with employees at risk of exposure to identify and implement new, safer devices into the workplace. Opinions on the adoption of safer techniques, along with identification of any new devices introduced to the workplace, should be documented in the Exposure Control Plan.

- **Universal precautions.** Employers must require employees to practice extreme, universal precautions when handling potentially infected materials. Employees must be trained to assume that all materials are infected with blood and/or other pathogens and protect themselves accordingly.

- **Engineering and work practice controls.** Controls should be implemented to address the use and proper handling of sharps disposal containers and needleless devices and proper hand hygiene. Document consultation with non-managerial healthcare workers who are responsible for direct patient care and are potentially exposed to injuries from contaminated sharps in identifying, evaluating and selecting effective engineering and work practice controls.

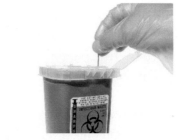

- **Housekeeping.** Employers must develop and implement housekeeping procedures, including decontamination procedures and the removal of regulated waste.

- **Personal protective equipment.** Employers must require employees to use personal protective equipment such as gloves, gowns, goggles, face shields and aprons. All equipment should be maintained, repaired and replaced at no cost to the employee.

- **Hepatitis B vaccination.** A part of the control plan is to offer the hepatitis B vaccination to every employee within ten days of being assigned to an area that exposes the employee to risk, at no cost to the employee. If the employee does not want to get the vaccine, the employer must have the employee sign a hepatitis B Vaccine declination statement, which must be kept with the employee's file.

Declination Statement

I understand that due to my occupational exposure to blood or other potentially infectious materials I may be at risk of acquiring hepatitis B virus (HBV) infection. I have been given the opportunity to be vaccinated with hepatitis B vaccine, at no charge to me; however, I decline hepatitis B vaccination at this time. I understand that by declining this vaccine I continue to be at risk of acquiring hepatitis B, a serious disease. If, in the future I continue to have occupational exposure to blood or other potentially infectious materials and I want to be vaccinated with hepatitis B vaccine, I can receive the vaccination series at no charge to me.

Employee Signature:_____

Date:_____

- **Exposure incident and post exposure evaluation follow-up.** Employees must be trained to report exposure incidents immediately, and employers must have procedures in place to address such incidents. Immediate and confidential medical evaluation and follow-up must be offered at no cost to any employee who reports an exposure. Lab tests must be conducted by an accredited lab (although an employee has the right to refuse an HIV test), and post-exposure prophylaxis and counseling must be offered to the employee.

The CDC emergency needlestick plan

- **Wash needlesticks and cuts with soap and water**
- **Flush splashes to the nose, mouth or skin with water**
- **Irrigate eyes with clean water, saline or sterile irrigants**
- **Seek immediate medical treatment**

- **Initial and annual training.** Employers must train employees on all BBP standard policies and procedures when they begin work or take on any job or activity that would expose them to risk. Annual training should be provided to address changes or updates to policies and procedures.

- **Records/documentation.** Employers must keep accurate and complete records of any work-related injuries or illnesses resulting from exposure to bloodborne pathogens. Employers should use these records to discover the causes, develop methods to prevent the incident from reoccurring and to monitor the effectiveness of new prevention procedures. Careful documentation of these efforts may reduce penalties if incompliance is found in an investigation.

Employers should create a schedule of how provisions of the BBP standard are to be implemented, including methods of compliance, HIV- and HBV-research laboratory and production facility requirements, hepatitis B vaccination and post-exposure evaluation and follow-up, communication of hazards to employees, and recordkeeping

The ECP must be reviewed and updated at least annually. It should be revised whenever tasks and procedures that affect occupational exposure are added or modified. It should also be updated to reflect new or revised employee positions with occupational exposure.

3.3.2.2 OSHA illness and injury recordkeeping

In order to evaluate the safety of a workplace, understand industry hazards, and implement worker protections to reduce and eliminate hazards, OSHA requires employers with 10 or more employees to keep a record of serious work-related injuries and illnesses, unless the employer is in a low-risk industry that is exempted.

Employers must record the following workplace injuries and illnesses:

- Work-related fatality

- Work-related injury or illness that results in loss of consciousness, days away from work, restricted work, or transfer to another job

- Work-related injury or illness requiring medical treatment beyond first aid

- Work-related diagnosed case of cancer, chronic irreversible diseases, fractured or cracked bones or teeth, and punctured eardrums

- OSHA has special recording criteria for work-related cases involving: needlesticks and sharps injuries; medical removal; hearing loss; and tuberculosis.

3.3.2.2.1 Immediate reporting for severe injuries:

Employers must notify OSHA when a worker is killed by reporting it within 8 hours. Workers that suffer a work-related hospitalization, amputation, or loss of an eye, must be reported within 24 hours.

3.3.2.2.2 Injury and illness forms:

Employers must track workplace injuries and illnesses on three separate forms:

1. **Injury and illness incident report (OSHA 301).** Employers must complete an Injury and Illness Incident Report within seven calendar days of learning that a recordable work-related injury or illness has occurred.

2. **Log of work-related injury and illness (OSHA 300).** Each recordable work-related injury or illness must also be recorded on the OSHA 300 Log within seven calendar days.

   Employees, a former employee, or an authorized employee representative have the right to access this document. In order to protect employee privacy, the words "privacy case" should recorded on the OSHA 300 Log instead of the employee's name for the following injuries and illnesses:

   - To an intimate body part or the reproductive system
   - Resulting from a sexual assault
   - Mental illnesses
   - HIV infection, hepatitis, or tuberculosis
   - Needlestick injuries and cuts contaminated with another person's blood or other potentially infectious material
   - ·Other illnesses, if the employee voluntarily requests that his or her name not be entered on the log

3. **Summary of work-related injuries and illnesses (OSHA 300A).** The OSHA 300A Form is an annual summary of the injuries and illnesses recorded on the OSHA 300 Log.

   The OSHA 300A Form for the previous year must be posted, in a common area where notices to employees are usually posted, no later than February 1 and kept in place until April 30. This posting is required, regardless of whether or not there have been any work-related injuries or illnesses.

OSHA Forms 301, 300, and 300A must be retained for five years. OSHA's Improve Tracking of Workplace Injuries and Illnesses rule requires electronic submission of workplace injuries and illnesses via the online Injury Tracking Application. The amended final rule issued on January 25, 2019 requires non-exempt employers to electronically submit OSHA Form 300A by March 2nd of the year after the calendar year covered by the form.

OSHA Recordkeeping FAQs

Do I need to report all workplace injuries with the OSHA 301 form?

No. You do not have to record an incident if it involves only: using non-prescription medications at nonprescription strength; administering tetanus immunizations; cleaning, flushing, or soaking wounds on the skin surface; using wound coverings, such as bandages, BandAids™, gauze pads, etc., or using SteriStrips™ or butterfly bandages. using hot or cold therapy; using any totally non-rigid means of support, such as elastic bandages, wraps, non-rigid back belts, etc.; using temporary immobilization devices while transporting an accident victim (splints, slings, neck collars, or back boards); drilling a fingernail or toenail to relieve pressure, or draining fluids from blisters; using eye patches; using simple irrigation or a cotton swab to remove foreign bodies not embedded in or adhered to the eye; using irrigation, tweezers, cotton swab or other simple means to remove splinters or foreign material from areas other than the eye; using finger guards; using massages; drinking fluids to relieve heat stress.

Do I need to record all cuts, lacerations, punctures, and scratches with the OSHA 301 form?

No. You must only record cuts, lacerations, punctures, and scratches that are work-related and involve contamination with another person's blood or other potentially infectious material. If the cut, laceration, or scratch involves a clean object, or a contaminant other than blood or other potentially infectious material, you need to record the case only if it meets one or more of the recording criteria in § 1904.7.1904.8(b)(3).

If I record an injury and the employee is later diagnosed with an infectious bloodborne disease, do I need to update the OSHA 300 Log?

Yes. You must update the classification of the case on the OSHA 300 Log if the case results in death, days away from work, restricted work, or job transfer. You must also update the description to identify the infectious disease and change the classification of the case from an injury to an illness.

3.3.3 Ionizing radiation standard

Any facility with x-rays or radioactive substances must comply with the Ionizing Radiation Standard (IRS). The standard includes these compliance components:

- Construction of the facility must be compliant with the ionizing radiation standard.
- A warning signal should be in place, **if** applicable.
- There must be a designated Radiation Security Officer who will be responsible for:
  - Scheduling equipment maintenance
  - Providing and maintaining personal protective equipment such as lead aprons
  - Providing radiation monitors
  - Minimizing any exposure risk to patients and employees
  - Testing a warning signal

3.3.3.1 Radiation exposure

The IRS standard directs employers to use the ALARA principle (As Low As Reasonably Achievable) when addressing radiation exposure levels. ALARA a work principle intended to protect the worker from unnecessary exposure to workplace hazards.

Radiation exposure is determined by these factors:

- Dose of "rads" (unit of absorbed radiation dose) received
- Duration of the exposure
- Distance from the radiation
- Type of shielding

In order to reduce the risk of radiation exposure, employers must perform ongoing radiation monitoring when working with x-ray or radioactive patients or materials using a personal monitoring device such as a film badge, double badge, ring badge or pocket dosimeter to identify and quantify the type of radiation exposure.

Measures that can help to protect employees and patients from radiation exposure include barrier walls with lead-plated glass windows; proper equipment maintenance; and other protective measures such as lead aprons and gloves and a warning sign.

3.3.3.2 Radiation Education and Information

The IRS standard requires employers to inform all employees working in or spending time in any part of a radiation area that radiation or radioactive materials are present.

Employers must provide information regarding the health risks associated with radiation exposure, such as acute dermatitis, erythema, chronic skin cancer or bone marrow damage.

Employers must also train employees on ways to minimize exposure, and measures to take in the event of a radiation emergency.

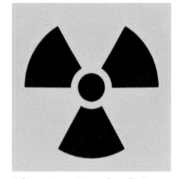

The international radiation symbol must be displayed in all radiation areas.

3.3.4 Exit routes standard

OSHA requires employers to establish exit routes in the event of an emergency. Exit routes standard components include:

- They must be permanent, unlocked and protected by a self-closing fire door.
- They must be separated from the rest of the facility by fire-resistant materials.
- They must be free of obstruction.
- There must be a sufficient number of exits (as codified by local fire code regulations).
- They must lead directly outside or to a street, walkway, refuge area, public way, or open space with access to the outside.

3.3.5 Electrical safety standard

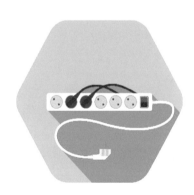

The OSHA Electrical Safety Standard (ESS) requires employers to develop an electrical safety plan to address: installation, routine maintenance, upgrades, troubleshooting and repair, moving and reinstallation and removal and disposal of all types of electrical equipment.

All electrical equipment be used as intended by the manufacturer, without any alterations. Employers should conduct regular inspections to ensure they are in compliance with the standard. Items to look for include:

- Damaged extension cords; NOTE: Extension cords should **not** be used to plug in equipment
- Damaged wall outlets
- Overloaded electrical circuits; this can be avoided with GFCI, fuses and circuit breakers
- Circuit breakers that do not have an on/off switch
- Improper grounding of equipment/circuitry—anything that is touched (light fixtures, light plates) should be grounded.

3.3.5.1 Electrical safety inspection log

An electrical safety plan should include a safety inspection log to record inspections and repairs to the following types of equipment:

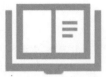

- Infrastructure equipment, including fire alarms, fire extinguishers, and waste removal equipment.

- Computer and security equipment used to access, store or maintain PHI and non-PHI, including work stations and handheld devices.

- Medical equipment, including any devices or equipment used to diagnose, treat or monitor patients.

- General office equipment, including appliances, copiers, shredders, fax machines etc.

3.3.6 Emergency action plan standard

The OSHA Emergency Action Plan (EAP) standard requires employers to develop a plan for fire and emergencies. The plan must include the following:

- Designated methods for reporting fire and emergencies (manual fire alarm, 911)
- Designation of a Safety Coordinator
- Evacuation policies, procedures and escape route assignments, including:
    - Who orders an evacuation
    - The actions that should be taken before evacuating the facility
    - The conditions that would trigger an evacuation
    - How to evacuate, including routes (exit diagrams)
    - The use of "fight or flee" portable fire extinguishers
    - Accounting for employees after an evacuation
    - Rescue and medical duties and the individuals responsible
    - Names/ job title of safety coordinator

3.3.7 Fire safety standard

Employers must design and implement a written fire safety plan that conforms to the OSHA Fire Safety standard.

All employees should be trained on the plan, which should include the following items:

- Identification of workplace fire hazards
- Steps to take in the event of a fire emergency, including escape routes/methods and the equipment that can be used for evacuation, if applicable

- A policy for the use of portable fire extinguishers; these extinguishers are not required, but if they are available, employees must receive hands-on training.

- Health warnings (and the corresponding SDSs) for any agents contained in fixed extinguishing systems used to detect fires, sound an alarm or spray water

- A back-up fire watch team if the fixed extinguishing team is out of service
- Include in EAP

- Emergency fire exits

- Emergency Action Plan

- A fire prevention plan to reduce the risk of fire and prevent the loss of life and property

- Employee smoking policies

- Alarm Systems (audible and visible)

3.3.8 Medical and first aid standard

The OSHA Medical and First Aid standard requires employers to train first aid personnel and to stock supplies that correspond to the hazards of the workplace in order to manage medical emergencies that may arise.

An employer must designate and train a person to provide first aid in the event of a medical emergency if the employer is not close to a clinic or hospital. The designated first aid care

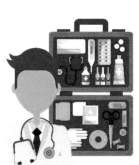

provider should be trained on how to conduct primary assessment and provide treatment, including use of first aid supplies and an automated external defibrillator. The designated first aid care provider should receive updates to training to keep accreditation current.

Employees must also be trained on the procedure to seek help for themselves or coworkers in a medical emergency.

OSHA does not have specific training or training requirements for managing non-life- or life-threatening emergencies. Employers must develop a program that is tailored to their needs, hazards, and proximity to medical care.

3.3.9 Personal protective equipment standard

OSHA requires employers to provide personal protective equipment (PPE) to employees in order to minimize exposure to workplace hazards.

To comply with the PPE standard, employers must:

- Identify and provide appropriate PPE

- Train employees on how to use and care for PPE, including what equipment to use/wear, when and how to use it, equipment limitations and equipment disposal

- Replace worn or damaged PPE

- Periodically review, update and evaluate the effectiveness of the PPE plan

- Ensure that the employees are wearing PPE whenever necessary

Workplace gloves

- **Replace gloves if they are tearing or deteriorating**

- **Provide non-latex gloves if an employee reports an allergy or sensitivity**

- **Never wash or re-use gloves**

- **When handling chemicals, refer to the SDS for the right glove type to wear**

3.4   Workplace Violence Prevention

Workplace violence is a serious issue, especially in healthcare facilities. In 2013 alone, over 25,000 occupational assault injuries occurred[6], most of which were in the health care and social services industries. OSHA responded by publishing guidelines on how to best prevent workplace violence. Although OSHA has no specific standards on the prevention of workplace violence, each employer has a general duty to keep employees safe in a hazard-free environment.

OSHA outlines the following five core elements for an effective workplace violence prevention program:

1. **Management commitment and employee participation**

It is essential that management show a strong commitment to the success of the workplace violence protection program and emphasize that aggressive or violent behavior is unacceptable and will have consequences. OSHA recommends creating a written workplace violence policy and posting it in publicly visible locations. In this way, management can clearly and unambiguously inform patients, visitors, employees, and others the conduct that is expected of them inside the healthcare facility. Clearly defined policies and procedures can also encourage employees to report violent incidents or other concerns and reassure them that their concerns will be addressed.

A joint committee of management and employees can ensure that all parties are participating, and all relevant knowledge and perspectives are heard. Committees can include representatives from all areas of the facility, including human resources, direct care staff,

---

[6] https://www.safetyandhealthmagazine.com/articles/12118-osha-updates-guidance-on-preventing-workplace-violence-in-health-care-social-services

security, legal departments, unions, and law enforcement. Research has shown that improved management commitment to a violence prevention program and employee engagement can lead to an increased perception of safety among staff.

2. Worksite analysis and hazard identification

Worksite analysis and hazard identification are key to the success of a workplace violence prevention program. Many factors can contribute to workplace violence in healthcare facilities. These risks include, but are not limited to:

- Working directly with people who have a history of violence, people who abuse drugs and alcohol, gang members, or distressed relatives or friends of patients or clients
- Lifting, moving, and transporting patients and clients
- Working alone in a facility or in patients' homes
- Poor environmental design of the workplace that may block employees' vision or interfere with their escape from a violent incident
- Poorly lit corridors, rooms, parking lots, and other areas
- Lack of a means of emergency communication
- Prevalence of firearms, knives, and other weapons among patients and their families and friends
- Working in neighborhoods with high crime rates

Some risks are more organizational, including but not limited to:

- Lack of facility policies and staff training for recognizing and managing escalating hostile and assaultive behaviors from patients, clients, visitors, or staff
- Working when understaffed in general- and especially during mealtimes, visiting hours, and night shifts
- High work turnover
- Inadequate security and mental health personnel on site
- Long waits for patients or clients and overcrowded, uncomfortable waiting rooms
- Unrestricted movement of the public in clinics and hospitals
- Perception that violence is tolerated, and victims will not be able to report the incident to police and/or press charges
- An overemphasis on customer satisfaction over staff safety

It is important for employees and employers to be cognizant of these and other risk factors and recognize them when they appear.

Worksite analysis includes reviewing records, procedures, and employee input. OSHA suggests that facilities review certain types of records to identify trends and risk factors including:

- Violence-related medical, safety, threat assessment, workers' compensation, and insurance records

- Logs of work-related injuries and illnesses, as required by OSHA (OSHA Forms 300 and 301)

- First reports of injury, incident/near-miss logs, and other incident reports, including police reports, general event logs, or daily logs

Worksite analysis could include employee surveys and questionnaires, patient surveys, focus groups with patients, and patient interviews. Finally, regular walkthrough assessments can help to identify and mitigate workplace hazards.

3. Hazard prevention and control

Once a review of the records and hazards has been completed, the next step is to work towards preventing and controlling the hazards that were identified. Prevention and control can minimize both risk and liability. There are two types of hazard controls as identified by OSHA: Engineering controls and administrative and work practice controls. The controls often work together to prevent risk, and they should both be tailored to the facility's needs and operations.

Engineering controls are physical changes to the workforce that either remove the hazard or create a barrier between the hazard and the employee. Examples include changing floor plans to make exits more accessible and/or improve sightlines for staff; improving lighting in remote areas or outdoor spaces for better visibility; installing mirrors; installing security technologies such as metal detectors, surveillance cameras, or panic buttons; and replacing furniture with heavier or fixed alternatives that cannot be easily used as weapons.

Administrative and work practice controls change the ways that employees perform their jobs and tasks in order to reduce the likelihood of violent incidents and to protect the staff, patients, and visitors. Examples include procedures and tools for assessing patients with regard to their potential for violent behavior; procedures for tracking and communicating information about a patient's behavior; special procedures for patients who have been violent in the past; adequate staffing on all units and shifts; training in de-escalation techniques, workplace safety, and trauma-informed care; and emergency procedures that prepare staff to know what to do in the case of an incident. Once these controls are in place, they must be periodically evaluated to ensure that they are doing enough to prevent or minimize hazards.

4. Safety and health training

Adequate training provides workers with information about how to recognize potential hazards and how protect themselves, their coworkers, and their patients. It can also help increase employees' confidence in their ability to handle violent situations.

Any worker who can reasonably be expected to interact with patients should receive training. Manager and supervisor training should provide them with the information needed to understand and execute their responsibilities in the event of an incident. Training programs should be customized specifically for the facility or for the unit within the facility, as each program would focus on the threats that the unit most commonly faces. A facility should give their employees frequent opportunities to practice the skills that they've learned in training.

Specific training topics as outlined by OSHA can include:

- A review of the facility's workplace violence prevention policies and procedures
- Policies and procedures for obtaining a patient's risk profile before admission
- Risk factors that cause or contribute to assaults
- Policies and procedures to assess and document patient or client behavioral changes
- Location, operation, and coverage of safety devices such as alarm systems, along with the required maintenance schedules and procedures
- Recognition of escalating behavior
- De-escalation techniques to prevent or defuse volatile situations
- Approaches to deal with aggressive behavior
- Proper use of safe rooms or areas where staff can find shelter from violence
- A standard response action plan for violent situations
- What to do in case of workplace violence
- Self-defense procedures
- Progressive behavior control methods
- Policies and procedures for reporting and recordkeeping
- Policies and procedures for getting medical care, counseling, workers' compensation, or legal assistance after a violent episode

Training programs should be repeated as often as needed. In high-risk situations, it may be advisable to have refresher training more often, for example, once a month. Training programs should be constantly evaluated and improved as the coordinator for the training assesses the content, method, and effectiveness of the program.

5. Recordkeeping and program evaluation

Recordkeeping and program evaluation assess the effectiveness of the program, identify hazards, and determine how the program could be continually improved. Regular reevaluation of policies and procedures will also help management stay informed and adapt to changing circumstances and needs.

Accurate reporting of incidents, hazards, training, and patient histories can help healthcare providers determine the extent of workplace violence issues, identify trends and patterns, evaluate methods of hazard control, and judge whether programs are working and/or need to be modified.

Clearly defined policies and procedures for reporting violent incidents is the key to effective reporting. Employees must not be retaliated against for voicing their concerns. OSHA prohibits discrimination against an employee for reporting a work-related injury or illness. Further, reporting procedures must protect employee and patient confidentiality.

According to OSHA, processes involved in a workplace violence prevention program evaluation usually include:

- Establishing a uniform definition of violence, reporting system, and regular review of reports

- Reviewing reports and minutes from staff meetings on safety and security issues

- Analyzing trends and rates in illnesses, injuries, or fatalities caused by violence relative to initial or "baseline" rates, and sharing data with management at all levels

- Measuring improvement based on lowering the frequency and severity of workplace violence

- Keeping up-to-date records of administrative and work practice changes to prevent workplace violence to evaluate how well they work

- Surveying workers before and after making job or worksite changes or installing security measures or new systems to evaluate their effectiveness

- Tracking recommendations through to completion

- Keeping abreast of new strategies available to prevent and respond to violence

- Surveying workers periodically to learn if they experience hostile situations at work

- Complying with OSHA and state requirements for recording and reporting injuries, illnesses, and fatalities

- Establishing an ongoing relationship with local law enforcement and educating them about the nature and challenges of working with potentially violent patients

- ·Requesting periodic law enforcement or outside consultant review of the worksite for recommendations on improving worker safety

Records that should be analyzed during program evaluation include:

- OSHA Log of Work-Related Injuries and Illnesses and Injury and Illness Incident Report (OSHA Forms 300 and 301)
- Medical reports of work injury, workers' compensation reports, and supervisors' reports for each recorded assault
- Records of incidents of abuse, reports filed by security personnel, and records of verbal attacks or aggressive behavior that may be threatening
- Information recorded in the charts of patients with a history of past violence, drug abuse, or criminal activity
- Documentation of minutes of safety meetings, records of hazard analyses, and corrective actions recommended and taken
- Records of all training programs, their attendees, and the qualifications of the trainers

Additional evaluation tips include:

- Using the same tools for re-evaluation as for the initial worksite assessment and hazard identification process, to allow for consistent data comparison.
- Working closely with the workplace violence prevention committee to learn what has worked in reducing violence or to learn about barriers that have been encountered.
- Examining only those incident reports that have been submitted since the last assessment took place, to avoid any overlap.

Documenting all assessments as well as all changes introduced based on the results.
Making sure to assess the quality and effectiveness of training programs rather than simply noting their presence.

3.5   OSHA Violations

Employers that fail to meet OSHA requirements may be issued citations for violations. The violations may carry recommended or mandatory penalties, which range from verbal notification to citations, fines, and even prison time for certain violations. The penalty depends on the size of the business, previous violations, and the company's good faith and willingness to cooperate during an OSHA investigation.

Below are the six classes of OSHA violations and corresponding penalties.

3.5.1 De minimis violations

The least serious class is a de minimis violation, which is a technical infraction that does not present a danger to workers and does not affect workplace safety or health.

Penalty: An OSHA inspector will not cite an employer for a de minimis violation. The employer will be informed about the violation and it will be recorded in the employer's file.

3.5.2 Other-than-serious violations

An other-than-serious violation is one that is related to workplace health and safety, but is unlikely to result in death or serious injury. Examples including failing to provide workers with copies of safety regulations or to post required documentation in work areas.

3.5.3 Serious violations

A serious violation is when an employer knows or should know about an issue that could cause serious injury or death and does nothing about it. An example is an employer who fails to ensure that employees who carry heavy loads wear steel-toe boots.

3.5.4 Willful violations

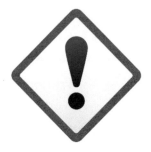

Willful violations are the most serious and carry the highest penalties. A willful violation is an intentional violation of OSHA rules or a blatant disregard for workplace health and safety. An example of a willful violation is the failure to protect workers from bloodborne pathogens.[7]

3.5.5 Repeated violations

As the name suggests, a repeated violation is when an employer is cited for a violation, and that same or a very similar violation is discovered during a subsequent inspection. Note: If the employer has formally contested the initial violation and has not yet received a final decision from OSHA, the employer cannot be cited for a repeated violation.

3.5.6 Failure-to-abate-prior violation

A failure-to-abate-prior violation is issued to an employer if it does not rectify the problems listed an OSHA citation by the date specified on the citation.

---

[7] https://www.osha.gov/news/newsreleases/region5/08112015

What did you learn? Discussion topics for Chapter 3

➢ Which employers are required to comply with OSHA requirements?

➢ What should an employer keep in mind when developing an OSHA compliance program?

➢ What are the nine OSHA standards that apply to the healthcare industry?

➢ What are the six steps for developing an effective Hazard Communication Program?

➢ Which OSHA violation is the most serious? What are the possible consequences for an individual citing for this class of violation?

Online Resources

"OSHA Forms for Recording Work-Related Injuries and Illness." Employers must record all work-related injuries, illnesses and deaths using these OSHA forms. https://www.osha.gov/recordkeeping/new-osha300form1-1-04-FormsOnly.pdf

"Job Safety and Health—It's the Law!" Employers must post this free workplace poster in a conspicuous place. https://www.osha.gov/Publications/poster.html

"OSHA QuickCard Hazard Communication Safety Data Sheets." This document summarizes the required format for Safety Data Sheets that chemical manufacturers, distributors or importers must use to communicate the hazards of hazardous chemical products. https://www.osha.gov/Publications/OSHA3493QuickCardSafetyDataSheet.pdf

"OSHA Brief—Hazard Communication Standard Safety Data Sheets." This document provides detailed information regarding the required for Safety Data Sheets that chemical manufacturers, distributors or importers must use to communicate the hazards of hazardous chemical products to downstream users. https://www.osha.gov/Publications/OSHA3514.pdf

"OSHA Fact Sheet—OSHA's Bloodborne Pathogens Standard." This document provides detailed information regarding the OSHA requirements for what employers must do to protect workers who are occupationally exposed to blood or other potentially infectious materials (OPIM). https://www.osha.gov/OshDoc/data_BloodborneFacts/bbfact01.pdf

"OSHA QuickCard Hazard Communication Standard Pictogram." This document summarizes the label pictograms that must be used to alert users of the chemical hazards to which they may be exposed. https://www.osha.gov/Publications/OSHA3491QuickCardPictogram.pdf

"OSHA Fact Sheet—Planning and Responding to Workplace Emergencies." This document summarizes the components of an effective safety and health management system for handling workplace emergencies. https://www.osha.gov/OshDoc/data_General_Facts/factsheet-workplaceemergencies.pdf

"Computer Workstation eTool." This checklist from the Department of Labor can be used to create a safe and comfortable computer workstation. It can also be used in conjunction with the purchasing guide checklist. https://www.osha.gov/SLTC/etools/computerworkstations/checklist_evaluation.html

"Workers' Rights." This publication provides a general overview of worker rights under the Occupational Safety and Health Act (OSH Act). https://www.osha.gov/Publications/osha3021.pdf

"Evacuation Plans and Procedures eTool." Use this online tool to develop a tailored emergency action plan. https://www.osha.gov/SLTC/etools/evacuation/expertsystem/emergencyplan.html

"OSHA Fact Sheet—Fire Safety in the Workplace." This document discusses employer requirements for training employees on workplace fire hazards and what to do in a fire emergency. https://www.osha.gov/ OshDoc/data_General_Facts/FireSafetyN.pdf

"Fire Prevention Plans." This OSHA regulation page describes the elements of a fire prevention plan. https://www.osha.gov/pls/oshaweb/owadisp.show_document?p_table=STANDARDS&p_id=12887

"Recording criteria for needlestick and sharps injuries." This OSHA regulation page describes the recordkeeping requirements for work-related needlestick injuries. https://www.osha.gov/pls/oshaweb/owadisp.show_document?p_table=STANDARDS&p_id=9639

"OSHA Fact Sheet—Updates to OSHA's Recordkeeping Rule: Who is Required to Keep Records and Who is Exempt." This document lists the industries required to prepare and maintain records of serious occupational injuries and illnesses using the OSHA 300 Log. https://www.osha.gov/recordkeeping2014/OSHA3746.pdf

"OSHA's Form 300 and 300A." This electronic document can be used to log and post a summary of work-related injuries and illnesses. https://www.osha.gov/recordkeeping/new-osha300form1-1-04-FormsOnly.pdf

"OSHA Hospital eTool: Clinical Services/Radiology." This OSHA resource considers the potential health hazards related to radiation exposure and possible solutions to minimize exposure. https://www.osha.gov/SLTC/etools/hospital/clinical/radiology/radiology.html#Radiation

"Design and construction requirements for exit routes." This OSHA regulation page provides design and construction requirements for exit routes in the event of an evacuation. https://www.osha.gov/pls/oshaweb/owadisp.show_document?p_table=STANDARDS&p_id=9724#1910.36(a)(3)

"OSHA Evacuation Plans and Procedures eTool." This OSHA resource provides information about the safe use of exit routes during an emergency, lighting and marking exit routes, fire retardant paints, exit routes during construction, repairs, or alterations, and employee alarm systems. https://www.osha.gov/ SLTC/etools/evacuation/egress.html

"OSHA Evacuation Plans and Procedures eTool; Emergency Action Plan." Employers can use this OSHA resource to generate a tailored Emergency Action Plan. https://www.osha.gov/ SLTC/etools/evacuation/ expertsystem/emergencyplan.html

"OSHA Best Practices Guide: Fundamentals of a Workplace First-Aid Program." This online guide provides a summary of the basic elements of a first-aid program in the workplace. https://www.osha.gov/Publications/OSHA3317first-aid.pdf

"OSHA Fact Sheet—Personal Protective Equipment (PPE) Reduces Exposure to Bloodborne Pathogens." This document provides information about selecting and disposing of PPE. https://www.osha.gov/OshDoc/data_BloodborneFacts/bbfact03.pdf

"Workplace Violence Prevention and Related goals." This OSHA article t illustrates how a workplace violence prevention program can complement and enhance your organization's strategies for compliance, accreditation, and quality of care. https://www.osha.gov/Publications/OSHA3828.pdf

"Guidelines for Preventing Workplace Violence for Healthcare and Social Service Workers." This publication provides a general overview of worker rights under OSHA. https://www.osha.gov/Publications/osha3148.pdf

"Caring for Our Caregivers—Preventing Workplace Violence: A Roadmap for Healthcare Facilities." OSHA developed this resource to assist healthcare employers and employees interested in establishing a workplace violence prevention program or strengthening an existing program. https://www.osha.gov/Publications/OSHA3827.pdf

Chapter 4

Federal Employment Laws

Overview

Federal laws prohibit employee discrimination in recruiting, hiring, job evaluations, promotion policies, training, compensation and disciplinary action. In this chapter, you will learn about the different federal employment laws that healthcare employers must comply with.

Chapter Outline

4.1   Federal anti-discrimination laws
4.2   Americans with Disabilities Act--Accommodations
4.3   Family and Medical Leave Act
4.4   Fair Labor Standards Act
4.5   Equal Employment Opportunity Commission
4.6   Workplace posters

Learning Objectives

After completing this chapter, you should be able to do the following:

✓   Name and describe the protected classes under Title VII, ADEA, GINA, and ADA.
✓   Explain how your organization can comply with the Americans with Disability Act.
✓   Understand and avoid direct and indirect discrimination in the workplace.
✓   Understand how to properly apply the provisions of the Family Medical Leave Act.
✓   Explain the Equal Opportunity Commission's role in protecting employee rights.

4.1   Federal Anti-Discrimination Laws

4.1.1 Overview

Federal anti-discrimination laws prohibit all employers from discriminating against employees or prospective employees who fall into "protected class" categories, such as age, gender, race, color, religion, sexual orientation, genetic information, and disabilities.

Employees and applicants are protected from negative treatment in the terms, conditions, and privileges in all areas of employment, including hiring and firing, discipline, pay and benefits, promotions and demotions, test and other selection criteria, work assignments and training, harassment, and retaliation.

4.1.1.1 Types of discrimination

Labor experts divide discrimination into two types: Direct discrimination and indirect discrimination.

Direct discrimination is when an individual who is part of a protected class is treated differently than similarly-situated employees. For example, an employer disciplines a female employee significantly more harshly than a male employee in the same or similar job.

Indirect discrimination refers to a policy or action that may appear to be neutral on the surface, but in fact has an adverse impact on a protected class. For example, an employer gives a written examination to potential hires that has a low pass rate for some minority groups. On its face, this looks like a neutral policy because all applicants are required to take the same exam. In practice, however, the exam adversely impacts a protected class that is more likely to fail it.

4.1.1.2 Harassment

Legally, harassment is defined as any unwelcome conduct that is based on an individual's membership in a protected class that creates a hostile or abusive working environment and/or becomes a condition of continued employment.

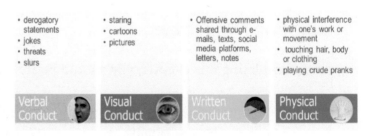

Who are potential harassers? A harasser could be someone from within the company, such as co-worker, supervisor, manager, or company executive. It could also be someone outside the company, such as a customer, patient, an independent contractor, or a vendor.

Harassment can occur in a number of different ways:

Verbal Conduct	**Someone makes derogatory statements, jokes, threats, slurs about an employee**
Visual Conduct	**Someone stares or shares offensive cartoons and pictures with an employee**
Written Conduct	**Someone shares offensive comments about an employee through e-mails, texts, social media platforms, letters, notes**
Physical Conduct	**Someone physically interferes with an employee's work or movement, such as touching hair, body or clothing or playing crude pranks**

 The Occupational Workplace Safety and Health Act (OSHA), also requires employers to provide employees with "safe and healthful" workplace environments. OSHA offers guidance and materials to develop a workplace violence prevention program. OSHA defines workplace violence as violent acts (including physical assaults and threats of assaults) directed toward persons at work or on duty.

4.1.1.3 Retaliation

Retaliation is another form of harassment. Under federal anti-discrimination laws, it is illegal to fire, demote, harass, or otherwise retaliate against an employee who opposes or complains about discrimination, or participates in an investigation of discrimination conducted by the employer, the Equal Employment Opportunity Commission (EEOC), or as part of a civil lawsuit.

4.1.1.4 Employer liability for discrimination

The consequences for an employer found guilty of discriminatory practices will depend on the person responsible for the discrimination and his or her role in the company.

There is strict liability if the discrimination was a "tangible employment action" carried out by a supervisor or manager, such as firing, promotion, undesirable work assignments, or benefits and compensation decisions.

An employer is liable for discrimination even if there was no tangible employment action, unless the employer used reasonable care to prevent and correct any harassment, **and** the victim failed to take advantage of preventive or corrective opportunities provided by the employer.

In the case of non-supervisory actions, an employer is liable if he or she knew, or should have known, about the harassment and did not take fast and appropriate action to correct the problem.

4.1.1.5 Legal remedies

Employers that are found guilty of discrimination or harassment can face steep penalties, and victims have multiple avenues for legal recourse available to them:

- Lost wages, such as salary and benefits
- Compensatory damages, which pay the victims for out-of-pocket costs that resulted from the discrimination, such as job searches, medical expenses, as well as for any mental harm suffered
- Punitive damages, used to punish an employer who has been found to have committed an especially malicious or reckless act of discrimination
- Attorney fees
- Court costs
- Reinstatement (getting back one's job)

Healthcare employers that are subject to the federal anti-discrimination laws are required to have a workplace free of discrimination, harassment and retaliation. There are four important anti-discrimination laws that healthcare employers must consider when developing a compliance program.

4.1.2 Title VII of the Civil Rights Act

Title VII applies to employers that have 15 or more employees. It prohibits discrimination in the workplace based on a recognized protected class. The classes covered by Title VII include:

Race	**Skin color, hair texture, or facial features associated with race**
Color	**Skin color and complexion**
Religion	**Religious beliefs; any aspect of religious practices or observances. Also includes the lack of religious beliefs, such as atheism and agnosticism**
National Origin	**Birthplace, ancestry, culture, accent, or linguistic characteristics**
Sex	**Gender, sexual harassment based on stereotyped expectations of behavior—this includes harassment based on sexual orientation, gender identity or transgender status. This category also includes unwelcome sexual advances, requests for sexual favors and other verbal, visual, physical or written conduct of a sexual nature.**

4.1.2.1 Preg Discrimination Act

Passed in 1978, The Pregnancy Discrimination Act amended Title VII to expand the scope of the protected class of "Sex" to pregnant women. The Act prohibits sex-based discrimination based on pregnancy, childbirth, and related medical conditions—including breastfeeding.

See Section 4.4.1 for more information about Affordable Care Act protections for breastfeeding employees.

4.1.3 Age Discrimination in Employment Act (ADEA)

The ADEA applies to employers with 20 or more employees. It prohibits the discrimination of certain applicants and employees 40 years of age or older based on age.

The Older Workers Benefit Protection Act (OWBPA) is an amendment to the ADEA. It was added to protect employees against age discrimination with regard to employee benefits, including life insurance, health insurance, employee benefits, pensions, retirement benefits, and other benefits provided by the employer.

The OWBPA also requires employers to follow certain rules when they ask employees to sign a "waiver of claims." This is a release that an employee signs agreeing not to sue his or her employer for age discrimination, in exchange for an incentive package to voluntarily quit his or her job. Under the OWBPA, the release must be "knowing and voluntary," which means it must be in writing and in plain English, and refer to the ADEA; it cannot misinform the employee or exaggerate the benefits the employee is receiving; and it cannot require the employee to waive rights or claims that come up after the employee signs the release.

Finally, the OWBPA protects employees in the event of layoffs. It requires employers to provide information about how the layoff decision was made, and the factors contributing to selection of employees affected by the layoff. This information gives employees the opportunity to determine whether age was a factor in the layoff.

4.1.4 Genetic Information Nondiscrimination Act (GINA)

GINA applies to employers with 15 or more employees. It prohibits discrimination based on genetic information.

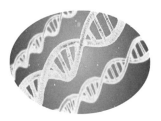

According to this Act, employers cannot request, purchase, or consider genetic test results about an employee, applicant or their family members.

Genetic information refers to any information about an employee's, an applicant's, or a family member's genetic test. This includes information about family medical history, defined as the manifestation of a disease or disorder in an individual's family members.

Under this Act, medical information that the employer has must be maintained in separate files and treated as a confidential medical record. It cannot be considered part of the employee's employment record. For healthcare providers, this is an important point. It means that a healthcare provider that is involved with the treatment of an employee cannot use that information for employment purposes.

4.1.5 Americans with Disabilities Act (ADA)

The ADA applies to employers with 15 or more employees. It prohibits discrimination of the following categories of individuals:

- Individuals with a physical or mental disability.
- Individuals who do not currently have a disability, but have a record of having a disability.
- Individuals who do not actually have a disability but are perceived as having one.

4.1.5.1 ADA definition of disability

The ADA uses a broad definition for disability, characterizing disability as "physical or mental impairment that substantially limits one or more major life activities." Major life activities include the following:

Caring for oneself	Standing	Breathing
Performing Manual Tasks	Sitting	Learning
Seeing	Reaching	Reading
Hearing	Major bodily functions	Concentrating
Eating	Lifting	Communicating
Sleeping	Bending	Interacting with others
Walking	Speaking	

Note that this list is not exhaustive. The ADA requires an individual assessment to determine whether a person has a disability.

Which conditions are **not** considered disabilities? According the ADA, conditions that last for only a few days or weeks, are not substantially limiting, and do not have a long-term effect on an individual's health are not considered disabilities. This includes short-term illnesses like the common cold and the flu, and injuries such as broken bones and sprains.

4.1.5.2 Disabilities recognized by the ADA

There are certain conditions that the ADA recognizes as disabilities. The conditions listed below immediately qualify as a disability.

Deafness	**Blindness**	**Intellectual disability**
Cancer	**Cerebral palsy**	**Diabetes**
Epilepsy	**HIV infection**	**Multiple sclerosis**
Muscular Dystrophy	**Autism**	**An impairment that is episodic or in remission**
Partially or completely missing limbs	**Mobility impairments requiring the use of a wheelchair**	**Major depressive disorder, bipolar disorder, post-traumatic stress disorder, obsessive compulsive disorder, schizophrenia**

Conditions that are episodic or in remission are still considered disabilities if it substantially limits major life activity when active, such as asthma, cancer, epilepsy, hypertension or diabetes.

4.1.5.3 Conditions not recognized as disabilities under the ADA

The conditions listed below are **not** considered to be impairments by the ADA:

Transvestism	**Transexualism**	**Pedophilia**
Exhibitionism	**Voyeurism**	**Gender identity disorders not resulting from physical impairments**
Other sexual behavior disorders	**Compulsive gambling**	**Kleptomania**
Pyromania	**Homosexuality**	**Bisexuality**
Psychoactive substance use disorders due to illegal drug use		

Note that although illegal drug use is not protected under the ADA, recovering drug addicts **are** covered under the ADA. This means that individuals addicted to drugs but are no longer using drugs illegally and are receiving treatment for drug addiction, or have been rehabilitated successfully are protected from discrimination by the ADA.

> **The ADA excludes transvestism, transsexualism, and gender-identity disorders not resulting from physical impairments. However, a Pennsylvania federal judge ruled in *Blatt v. Cabela's Retail Inc.* (E.D. Pa. May 18, 2017) that gender dysphoria would not be excluded from ADA because the condition goes beyond merely identifying with a different gender and is characterized by clinically significant stress and other impairments that may be disabling.**

4.2   Americans with Disabilities Act—Accommodations

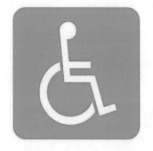

The ADA requires an employer to provide "reasonable accommodations for a known mental or physical limitation of a qualified individual with a disability."

In order to know whether an employee is eligible for an accommodation under the ADA, the employer must first determine whether the individual is qualified. Under the ADA, a qualified individual is someone who can perform the essential functions of the job with or without reasonable accommodation. (Essential functions refer to the basic job duties that an employee must perform; they do not include marginal job functions.)

4.2.1 Accommodations—Definition

The ADA defines a reasonable accommodation as any change or adjustment to a job or work environment that enables the individual to access equal employment opportunities.

Only those employees with a current or "record" of disability are eligible for accommodations. Employees that are "regarded as" having a disability but do not have one are **not** eligible for accommodations because they don't need them.

4.2.2 Determining appropriate accommodations

The employer and the employee must work together to determine whether the employee is a qualified individual who is eligible for accommodations, and to identify the appropriate accommodations. This interactive process should include these steps:

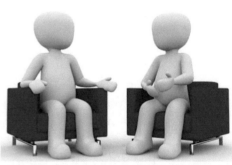

- Determine what the employee's limitations are due to the disability.
- Identify potential reasonable accommodations that could overcome those limitations. Note that an employee does not have to provide requested accommodations, but rather reasonable accommodations.

- Document the interactive process. Documentation should be done by the employer.

4.2.3 Medical documentation

An employer may need additional information to confirm that the employee is disabled and requires accommodations. In those cases, the employer is allowed to ask the employee to provide medical documentation to substantiate the disability. If the employer finds that the information provided by the employee is not sufficient, the employer can require the employee to see a healthcare professional. The employer must cover the cost of that visit.

 The employer cannot ask an employee or healthcare professional to provide medical documentation that is not related to the disability. Any medical information provided to the employer must be maintained in a separate employee file and treated as a confidential medical record.

What do accommodations look like?

Accommodations vary depending on the needs of the individual applicant or employee. The decision about which accommodation should be made on a case-by-case basis and take into account the nature and extent of the disability, as well as the conditions of the job.

Here are some examples of accommodations that employers may consider when working with a disabled applicant or employee:

- Making existing facilities (lunchrooms, restrooms, etc) accessible to disabled persons
- Job restructuring
- Modifying work schedules
- Reassignment to a vacant position
- Acquiring/modifying equipment or devices
- Modifying examinations, training materials, or policies
- Providing qualified readers or interpreters
- Modifying a job application process to include qualified disabled applicants
- Making employer provided transportation accessible
- Providing reserved parking spaces
- Providing additional unpaid leave for necessary treatment

4.2.4 Employer defenses for not providing accommodations

An employer may claim that it is not possible to provide accommodations to an employee with a disability. The ADA allows employers to decline to make accommodations if they will cause the employer undue hardship or if the disabled employee presents a direct threat to him/herself and/or other employees.

An **undue hardship** would be an accommodation that would require significant expense or be very difficult to execute. Factors for determining undue hardship include the nature and cost of the accommodation, the overall financial resources and operations of the employer, and the impact the accommodation would have on the operation of the business. A larger employer would typically be expected to make accommodations requiring greater effort or expense than would be required of a smaller employer.

A **direct threat** is when an individual's presence in the workplace poses a significant risk of substantial harm to the health or safety to him/herself or to others that cannot be eliminated or reduced by reasonable accommodation. An employer must substantiate a claim of a direct threat with medical evidence.

4.2.5 Employer retaliation

Just as an employer cannot retaliate against an employee who makes a discrimination claim, an employer cannot retaliate against an employee who invokes his or her rights under the ADA and requests an accommodation. Employees have the right to claim a disability and request that an employer engage in an interactive process to determine appropriate accommodations without having to fear for his or her job.

4.3 Family and Medical Leave Act

The Family and Medical Leave Act (FMLA) applies to private employers with 50 or more employees, as well as all public agencies. It is enforced by the Department of Labor (DOL). To be eligible for FMLA, an employee must have worked at least 12 months in total, and must have worked at least 1,250 hours over the past 12-month period.

> If a company has multiple locations, the FMLA applies if the company has 50 or more employees within a 75-mile radius. For example, if you have 3 locations and they are 20 miles apart from each other with 30 employees at each location, you must comply with the FMLA.

4.3.1 Protections

Under the FMLA, employees are entitled to 12 weeks of unpaid, job-protected leave in a 12-month period. The leave can be used for the birth or adoption of a child, or due to a serious health condition of the employee or the employee's family member.
Serious health conditions include the following:

- An illness that requires inpatient care or continuing treatment by a healthcare provider, with an incapacity lasting more than three consecutive days.

- Leave for pregnancy/prenatal care.

- Chronic serious health conditions, such as asthma or diabetes.

- Permanent or long-term conditions, such as Alzheimer's disease, strokes, and terminal illnesses.

Serious health conditions must be determined on a case-by-case basis. Temporary conditions (for example, colds, influenza) are **not** considered serious health conditions.

4.3.2 Military leave

FMLA also includes provisions for military leave in the form of qualifying exigency leave and military caregiver leave.

Eligible employees may take up to 12 weeks of unpaid, job-protected FMLA leave in a 12-month period for a qualifying exigency that arises from the foreign deployment of the employee's spouse, son, daughter, or parent with the Armed Forces. Qualifying exigency leave includes the following:

- Up to seven days of leave to address any issue that arises from a military family member's short-notice deployment (deployment within seven or less days of notice)

- To attend military events and related activities (official ceremonies, programs, events and informational briefings, or family support or assistance programs sponsored by the military, military service organizations, or the American Red Cross that are related to deployment)

- For childcare and related activities (arranging for alternative childcare, providing childcare on a non-routine, urgent, immediate need basis, enrolling in or transferring a child to a new school or day care facility)

- To care for the military family member's parent who is incapable of self-care (arranging for alternative care, providing care on a non-routine, urgent, immediate need basis, admitting or transferring a parent to a new care facility, and attending certain meetings with staff at a care facility)

- To make/update financial and legal arrangements (preparing and executing financial and healthcare powers of attorney, enrolling in the Defense Enrollment Eligibility Reporting System, or obtaining military identification cards)

- To attend counseling for the employee, the military family member, or the child of the military family member

- Up to 15 calendar days of leave to spend time with a military family member who is on short-term, temporary rest and recuperation leave during deployment

- For post-deployment activities (attending arrival ceremonies, reintegration briefings and events, and other official ceremonies or programs sponsored by the military, and addressing issues arising from the death of a military member, including attending the funeral)

- For any other event that the employee and employer agree is a qualifying exigency

FMLA allows eligible employees to take leave to care for a service member with a serious injury or illness if the employee is the service member's spouse, son, daughter, parent or next of kin. For this type of leave, employees are allowed up to 26 weeks of unpaid, job-protected leave during a single 12-month period.

4.3.2.1 Uniformed Services Employment and Reemployment Rights Act (USERRA)

USERRA provides military leave for those employees who serve in the U.S. military, and provides job protection for when an employee returns from military duty. It applies to all employees, regardless of whether the employer is public or private, and regardless of the number of employees.

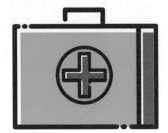

The Act also prohibits discrimination based on past, present or future military service.

4.3.3 Maintenance of health benefits under the FMLA

The FMLA requires employers to continue an employee's health insurance coverage during a leave period, so long as the employee makes his or her required insurance contribution.

4.3.4 Employee notice requirements and medical certification

In order to take leave under the FMLA, an employee must give the employer appropriate notice and provide information that supports the claim of a serious health condition. The employee must also provide the probable length of the absence.

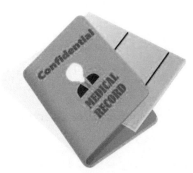

An employee does not have to specifically ask for FMLA leave if it is the first leave request. However, the employee **does** need to provide enough information so that the employer understands that the leave may be covered by the FMLA. If the employee is already approved for leave under the FMLA and needs to extend the leave, the employee must explicitly mention that he or she is on FMLA and the condition. Otherwise, the employer might not have enough information to know that the leave is covered by the FMLA.

The employer needs to determine whether the employee's situation qualifies for FMLA leave. To do that, the employer may require the employee to submit medical certification in order to confirm that the leave is covered by the FMLA.

The employer can contact the healthcare provider to clarify information regarding the health condition, or to authenticate the medical certification, after giving the employee the chance to correct any deficiencies. Contact with the healthcare provider may be made by the human resources department, a leave administrator or a manager. The employee's direct supervisor may **not** be the one to contact the healthcare provider.

Clarification can mean any number of things, from not being able to read the handwriting on a document to understand the meaning of a response. Authentication refers to asking the healthcare provider to confirm that the information is correct and was issued by the provider who signed the certification.

An employer must obtain a HIPAA authorization from the employee when seeking clarification of the medical documentation. If the employee refuses to sign a HIPAA release, and refuses to provide clarification regarding the medical information, the employer may deny leave under the FMLA. (A HIPAA release is not needed to authenticate a medical certification because the content of the certification is not being discussed).

If the employer is not convinced that the medical certification supports leave under the FMLA, the employer can request a second medical opinion from a healthcare provider of its choice and at its own expense. If the second opinion differs from the first, the employer and employee must mutually agree on a healthcare provider for a third opinion. The third opinion is final and binding.

Medical certification documents must be maintained in separate employee files and treated as confidential medical records.

4.3.5 Employer notice

Once an employer learns that an employee needs to take FMLA leave, the employer must provide the employee with three notices:

Eligibility Notice. This notice confirms that the employee is eligible for leave under the FMLA because he or she has been with the company for at least 12 months, has worked the minimum number of hours, and the company is covered by the FMLA.

Rights and Responsibility Notice: This notice provides information about the employee's obligations for using the FMLA.

Designation Notice: This notifies the employee whether the requested leave qualifies under the FMLA. Once the employer has enough information to determine whether the leave qualifies, it must notify the employee within five days.

The eligibility notice and rights and responsibility notice are usually provided together within five days of the employee's request for FMLA leave, or when the employer learns that an employee's leave may qualify for FMLA.

4.3.6 Returning to work

When an employee comes back to work after being on FMLA leave, he or she is entitled to resume his or her original job, or an equivalent job with equivalent pay, benefits and other employment terms and conditions. An equivalent job must have the same or substantially similar duties, responsibilities, skill requirements and authority.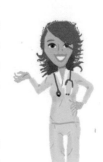

If the employee was on leave for his or her own serious health condition, the employer may require him or her to obtain a fitness for duty certification from a healthcare provider before returning to work.

4.3.7 Interference and retaliation

As with other employment protection rights, it is unlawful to interfere or retaliate against an employee who exercises or attempts to exercise their FMLA rights. An employer cannot refuse to authorize leave without determining whether the employee qualifies, and cannot discourage an employee from taking FMLA leave. Likewise, an employer cannot use the fact that an employee has taken FMLA leave against him or her, for example in hiring, promotion or disciplinary actions or decisions.

4.3.7.1 Legal remedies

If an employee demonstrates that he or she suffered interference or retaliation as a result of exercising or trying to exercise FMLA rights, he or she may be eligible for these legal remedies:

- Lost wages
- Damages for an employer's willful violations (employee damages are doubled)
- Attorney fees
- Court costs
- Reinstatement to a former position

4.4 Fair Labor Standards Act

The Fair Labor Standards Act (FLSA) is enforced by the Department of Labor and applies to any employer with annual gross sales of $500,000 or more, **or** to any employer that engages in interstate commerce. These broad requirements mean that most employers must comply with the FLSA.

The FLSA sets minimum wages and overtime pay requirements. It requires employers to keep detailed wage and hour records, sets hour/shift restrictions, and establishes occupational standards for minors.

4.4.1 FLSA and the Patient Protection and Affordable Care Act

The Patient Protection and Affordable Care Act (ACA) amended the FLSA on the day the ACA was signed in March of 2010 to address the needs of breastfeeding employees.

Breastfeeding employees are protected from discrimination under Title VII's Pregnancy Discrimination Act (See Section 4.1.2.1). The amended FLSA added protections by requiring employers to provide break times and suitable locations for breastfeeding activities.

The ACA amendment to the FLSA requires employers to provide reasonable break times for employees who are breastfeeding infants. Employees are eligible for breastfeeding breaks for one year after the birth of the child.

Under the amendment, the employer is also required to provide a space for breastfeeding purposes—other than a bathroom—that is shielded from view and free from intrusion from coworkers and the public.

4.4.2 FLSA and the Equal Pay Act

The Equal Pay Act (EPA) also amended the FLSA to provide protections to both men and women from pay discrimination based on gender.

The EPA requires employers to equally compensate men and women for jobs requiring equal skill, equal effort, equal responsibility and having similar working conditions.

All forms of pay are covered by the EPA: Salary, overtime pay, bonuses, stock options, profit-sharing, and any other benefits provided by the employer.

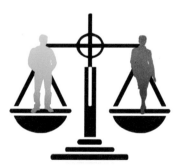

The EPA permits pay differentials that are based on seniority, merit, quantity or quality of production, or a factor other than gender. These are known as "affirmative defenses." If an employee claims pay discrimination under the EPA, the employer must be able to clearly demonstrate an affirmative defense reason for the differential.

Pay discrimination based on gender can also be a claim for sex-based discrimination under Title VII (See Section 4.1.2).

4.5 Equal Employment Opportunity Commission

The Equal Employer Opportunity Commission (EEOC) is the federal agency responsible for enforcing the federal non-discrimination laws discussed in Section 4.1, as well as the Equal Pay Act:

- Title VII of the Civil Rights Act
- The Age Discrimination in Employment Act
- The Americans with Disability Act
- The Genetic Information Nondiscrimination Act
- The Equal Pay Act

The EEOC issues regulations that implement the federal workplace anti-discrimination laws, which can be found in the Code of Federal Regulations (CFR).

4.5.1 EEOC investigations

If an individual believes that his or her rights protected under a federal anti-discrimination act (not including the Equal Pay Act) have been violated and wishes to pursue legal action, the first step is to a file a "charge of discrimination" with the EEOC. An individual must file this charge before filing a job discrimination lawsuit against an employer.

Complaints made under state discrimination laws do not have to be filed with the EEOC. Depending on the state, an individual may file with a similar state agency or may directly file a lawsuit.

If the EEOC decides to investigate a discrimination charge, it will work to determine whether there is reasonable cause to believe that discrimination occurred. The EEOC will request a written position statement from the employer, request additional documentation and may conduct interviews.

If there is a finding of discrimination, the EEOC may arrange for mediation between the employer and the individual to settle the matter. The EEOC also has the authority to file a federal discrimination lawsuit on behalf of the individual.

When the EEOC completes the investigation, or if it decides to dismiss the charge, it will issue a right-to-sue letter. This letter allows the individual to proceed with a federal lawsuit which must be filed within ninety days of receiving the letter from the EEOC.

4.6   Workplace Posters

Healthcare employers (like all employers) are required by law to hang federal posters prominently in the workplace to notify employees and job applicants of their rights regarding such topics as the minimum wage, health and safety, and other important labor laws. The Department of Labor provides free electronic copies of the required posters and some of the posters are available in languages other than English.

4.6.1 Posters for employees and applicants

The following posters must be prominently displayed where they can be readily seen by both employees and job applicants.

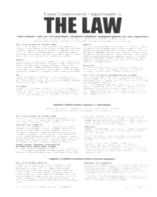

EEO is The Law

The EEO is the Law poster is prepared by the EEOC and summarizes the laws that it enforces. It explains how individuals can file a complaint with the EEOC.

https://www1.eeoc.gov/employers/poster.cfm

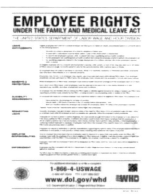

Employee Rights under the FMLA

The Family and Medical Leave Act poster must be posted by every employer subject to the FMLA even if there are no FML-eligible employees at the time. This poster notifies employees of their rights under the FMLA act.

https://www.dol.gov/whd/regs/compliance/posters/fmlaen.pdf

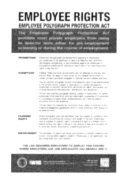

Employee Rights under the EPPA

The Employee Polygraph Protection Act poster informs individuals that employers cannot lie detector tests for pre-employment screening of job applicants or for testing current employees. All private employers must display this poster.

https://www.dol.gov/whd/regs/compliance/posters/eppac.pdf

4.6.2 Posters for employees

The following posters must be prominently displayed where they can be readily seen by employees only (not job applicants).

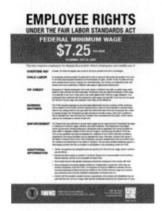

Employee Rights under the FLSA: Minimum Wage

Every employer subject to the FLSA's minimum wage provisions is required to display the FLSA poster which notifies employees of the law's requirements.

https://www.dol.gov/whd/regs/compliance/posters/flsa.htm

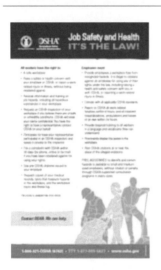

OSHA Job Safety and Health: It's the Law

The OSHA poster informs workers of the law's requirements under OSHA, including the right to work in a safe place. All private sector employers are required to display this poster.

https://www.osha.gov/Publications/poster.html

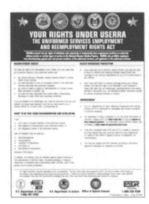

Your Rights Under USERRA

All employers are required to display the Uniformed Services Employment and Reemployment Rights Act poster, which informs employees that returning service members are entitled to receive all rights and benefits of employment that they would have obtained if they had been continuously employed.

https://www.dol.gov/vets/programs/userra/poster.htm

FEDERAL RECORD RETENTION PERIODS

Healthcare providers have enough documentation to keep track of when it comes to patients and their medical records. But retaining employment related documents is equally important. Here are the common employment records that need to be maintained based on federal requirements.

HIRING RECORDS
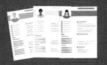

Including job applications, job advertisements / openings, resumes, failure to hire, employment tests, promotions, training programs, overtime work opportunities

1 year

PAYROLL

Or other records containing name, address, date of birth, occupation, rate of pay, and weekly compensation

3 years

EMPLOYEE MEDICAL RECORDS

Excludes a) health insurance claims records; b) first-aid records made onsite by a non-physician of one-time treatment and later observations that did not involve medical treatment; c) medical records of employees who have worked for less than 1 year if they are provided to the employee at end of employment

Duration of employment plus 30 years

LEAVE RECORDS

Dates/hours of FMLA leave, notices, leave policies, records of any dispute regarding leave

3 years

BASIC EMPLOYMENT AND EARNING RECORDS

Time cards, wage rate tables, work and time schedules, and records of additions to or deductions from wages

2 years

PERSONNEL RECORDS

Including requests for reasonable accommodation, job applications, hiring, promotion, demotion, transfer, lay-off or termination, rates of pay or other terms of compensation, and selection for training or apprenticeship

1 year

EMPLOYEE BENEFIT PLANS

Including pension and insurance plans, seniority and merit systems and merit systems

1 year

PAYMENT RECORDS
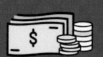

Any records relating to payment of wages, wage rates, job evaluations, job descriptions, merit or seniority systems, collective bargaining agreements, description of practices or other matters which describe or explain the basis for payment of any wage differential to employees of the opposite sex in the same establishment

2 years

FORM 1-9

Employment Eligibility Verification

3 years

EMPLOYEE EXPOSURE RECORDS

30 years

OSHA 300 LOG

Privacy case list (if any), annual summary, and OSHA 301 Incident Report forms

5 years

For more information view the blog article:
https://1sthcc.com/how-to-comply-with-federal-recordkeeping-requirements/

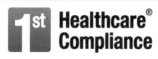

What did you learn? Discussion topics for Chapter 4

➤ Healthcare employers that are subject to the federal anti-discrimination laws are required to have a workplace free of discrimination, harassment and retaliation. What does creating a discrimination-free workplace involve?

➤ What process must be used to determine whether a disabled employee requires an accommodation, and what a reasonable accommodation could be?

➤ When do healthcare employers subject to the FMLA have to provide unpaid time off? What is the process for determining FMLA-eligibility?

➤ How do FLSA regulations impact healthcare employers with regard to wage and hour, overtime, child labor, record keeping, breastfeeding protections and equal pay?

➤ Both FLSA and FMLA are enforced by the Department of Labor. Which federal agency is responsible for enforcing the federal anti-discrimination laws (Title VII, ADEA, ADA, GINA, EPA)? What are the possible penalties an employer could incur for violating these laws?

➤ Which federal posters must be prominently displayed in the workplace in order to notify employees and job applicants of their rights?

Online Resources

"USEEOC Recordkeeping Requirements." This document explains the recordkeeping requirements of the Equal Employment Opportunity Commission and best practices for recordkeeping in the event a charge is filed. https://www1.eeoc.gov//employers/recordkeeping.cfm?renderforprint=1

"EEOC Age Discrimination Fact Sheet." This document explains the protections afforded individuals by the Age Discrimination in Employment ACT (ADEA). https://www.eeoc.gov/eeoc/publications/upload/age.pdf

"EEOC Equal Pay Fact Sheet." This document explains employee rights regarding equal pay, and the laws protecting those rights. https://www.eeoc.gov/eeoc/publications/upload/fs-epa.pdf

"EEOC Pregnancy Discrimination Fact Sheet." This document explains the protections afforded individuals by the Pregnancy Discrimination in Employment ACT (PDA). https://www.eeoc.gov/eeoc/publications/upload/fs-preg.pdf

"EEOC Sexual Harassment Fact Sheet." This document explains the protections afforded individuals by Title VII. https://www.eeoc.gov/eeoc/publications/upload/fs-sex.pdf

"The Employer's Guide to the Family and Medical Leave Act." This guide from the Department of Labor provides employers with information about the FMLA and the certification process. https://www.dol. gov/whd/fmla/employerguide.pdf

"Fact Sheet #73: Break Time for Nursing Mothers." This document provides general information on the break time requirement for nursing mothers in the Patient Protection and Affordable Care Act ("PPACA"). https://www.dol.gov/whd/regs/compliance/whdfs73.pdf

"FMLA: Fact Sheets." This webpage form the US Department of Labor website provides links to fact sheets with information about the protections and employer requirements of the FMLA, including Military Family Leave. https://www.dol.gov/whd/fmla/fact_sheets.htm

"FMLA: Forms." This webpage form the US Department of Labor website provides links to forms related to the FMLA. https://www.dol.gov/whd/fmla/forms.htm

"Handy Reference Guide to the Fair Labor Standards Act." This guide from the US Department of Labor provides an overview of the fair labor standards established by the Act regarding minimum wage, overtime pay, recordkeeping, and child labor standards affecting full-time and part-time workers in the private sector and in federal, state, and local governments. https://www.dol.gov/whd/regs/compliance/ wh1282.pdf

"Fact Sheet #36: Employee Polygraph Protection Act of 1988." This document provides general information about employee protections from the use of lie detector tests either for pre-employment screening or during the course of employment. https://www.dol.gov/whd/regs/compliance/whdfs36.pdf

Made in United States
Troutdale, OR
01/19/2024